Daniel Lee
Robert O'Gorman
Editors

Social Work and Divinity

Social Work and Divinity has been co-published simultaneously as *Journal of Religion & Spirituality in Social Work: Social Thought*, Volume 24, Numbers 1/2 2005.

Pre-publication REVIEWS, COMMENTARIES, EVALUATIONS . . .

"DIVERSE, FASCINATING, AND THOUGHT-PROVOKING. . . . Explores theoretical and practical aspects of dual degree programs and other structures for relating the two professions. It will help to nourish the transitional space between social work and divinity. With chapters ranging from conceptual to programmatic to empirical, the collection seems especially enriching for boundary spanners who have feet in both camps but who often work at the boundary alone."

Terry A. Wolfer, PhD
Associate Professor
College of Social Work
University of South Carolina

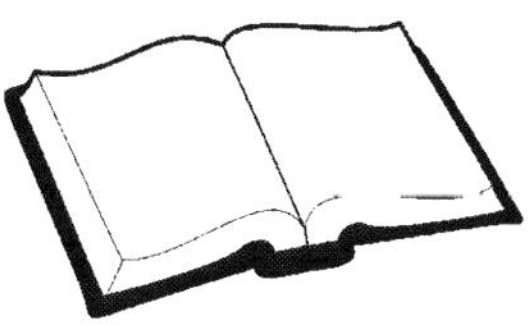

More pre-publication
REVIEWS, COMMENTARIES, EVALUATIONS . . .

"COMPREHENSIVE AND MULTI-DIMENSIONAL. . . . A delightfully refreshing and desperately essential compendium of interlocking discussions by distinguished scholars and practitioners. . . . A meaningful and inspirational call to action for university and seminary curricula to open their eyes, minds, hearts, and educational programs to embrace never-before conceptualized or practiced operational models of sharing information and coordination/integration strategies and techniques."

William D. Eldridge, PhD
Associate Professor and Psychotherapist
College of Social Work
The Ohio State University, Columbus

THSWPP

THPP

The Haworth Social Work Practice Press
The Haworth Pastoral Press
Imprints of The Haworth Press, Inc.

New York • London • Victoria (AU)
www.HaworthPress.com

Social Work and Divinity

Social Work and Divinity has been co-published simultaneously as *Journal of Religion & Spirituality in Social Work: Social Thought*, Volume 24, Numbers 1/2 2005.

The Journal of Religion & Spirituality in Social Work™ Monographic "Separates" (formerly *Social Thought: Journal of Religion in the Social Services*)*

Below is a list of "separates," which in serials librarianship means a special issue simultaneously published as a special journal issue or double-issue *and* as a "separate" hardbound monograph. (This is a format which we also call a "DocuSerial.")

"Separates" are published because specialized libraries or professionals may wish to purchase a specific thematic issue by itself in a format which can be separately cataloged and shelved, as opposed to purchasing the journal on an on-going basis. Faculty members may also more easily consider a "separate" for classroom adoption.

"Separates" are carefully classified separately with the major book jobbers so that the journal tie-in can be noted on new book order slips to avoid duplicate purchasing.

You may wish to visit Haworth's website at . . .

http://www.HaworthPress.com

. . . to search our online catalog for complete tables of contents of these separates and related publications.

You may also call 1-800-HAWORTH (outside US/Canada: 607-722-5857), or Fax 1-800-895-0582 (outside US/Canada: 607-771-0012), or e-mail at:

docdelivery@haworthpress.com

Social Work and Divinity, edited by Daniel Lee, DSW, and Robert O'Gorman, PhD (Vol. 24, No. 1/2, 2005). *"Diverse, fascinating, and thought-provoking. . . . Explores theoretical and practical aspects of dual degree programs and other structures for relating the two professions. It will help nourish the transitional space between social work and divinity. With chapters ranging from conceptual to programmatic to empirical, the collection seems especially enriching for boundary spanners who have feet in both camps but who often work at the boundary alone." (Terry A. Wolfer, PhD, Associate Professor, College of Social Work, University of South Carolina)*

Criminal Justice: Retribution vs. Restoration, edited by Eleanor Hannon Judah, DSW, ACSW, and Rev. Michael Bryant, PhD (Vol. 23, No. 1/2, 2004). *"Timely and necessary. . . . Of interest to students of social, economic, and behavioral sciences, philosophy, theology, and cultural history, as well as to the general public. As a student and teacher of social policy, social justice, and human development. I find this book thought provoking andI will recommend it to my students." (David G. Gil, DSW, Professor of Social Policy, Heller School for Social Policy and Management, Brandeis University)*

Practicing Social Justice,* edited by John J. Stretch, PhD, MBA, ACSW, LCSW, Ellen M. Burkemper, PhD, LCSW, MFT, William J. Hutchison, PhD, and Jan Wilson, ACSW, LCSW (Vol. 22, No. 2/3, 2003). *"I highly recommend this important edited work to practitioners, academics, and students majoring in the human services and related fields. . . . Fills an important void in the area of social justice and related issues. . . . Offers a detailed analysis of numerous social justice issues." (John T. Pardeck, PhD, LCSW, Editor,* Journal of Social Work in Disability and Rehabilitation*)*

Issues in Global Aging,* edited by Frederick L. Ahearn, Jr., DSW (Vol. 20, No. 3/4, 2001). *"Fine scholarship . . . very useful. Ahearn has assembled a fine cohort of experts on aging who address various issues. The first section approaches them from the western industrial model perspective, but also provides an example of an Islamic traditional approach. The second section deals less with formal religiosity than with issues of spiritual transcendence in older persons. A balanced portrait of the aged as people rather than statistics." (Charles Guzzetta, EdD, Professor, Hunter College, City University of New York)*

Transpersonal Perspectives on Spirituality in Social Work,* edited by Edward R. Canda, PhD, and Elizabeth D. Smith, DSW (Vol. 20, No. ½, 2001). *"Comprehensive . . . provides theoretical and practice-oriented studies on the emerging field of transpersonal social work. The writing is both scholarly and relevant to practice. Of interest to scholars, practitioners, and students alike." (John R Graham, PhD, RSW, Associate Professor, Faculty of Social Work, University of Calgary, Alberta, Canada)*

Raising Our Children Out of Poverty,* edited by John J. Stretch, PhD, Maria Bartlett, PhD, William J. Hutchison, PhD, Susan A. Taylor, PhD, and Jan Wilson, MSW (Vol. 19, No. 2, 1999). *This book shows what can be done at the national and local community levels to raise children out of poverty by strengthening families, communities, and social services.*

Postmodernism, Religion and the Future of Social Work,* edited by Roland G. Meinert, PhD, John T. Pardeck, PhD, and John W. Murphy, PhD (Vol. 18, No. 3, 1998). *"Critically important for social work as it attempts to effectively respond to its increasingly complex roles and demands. . . . A book worth owning and studying." (John M. Herrick, PhD, Acting Director, School of Social Work, Michigan State University, East Lansing, Michigan)*

Spirituality in Social Work: New Directions,* edited by Edward R. Canda, PhD (Vol. 18, No. 2, 1998). *"Provides interesting insights and references for those who seek to develop curricula responsive to the spiritual challenges confronting our profession and the populations we serve." (Au-Deane S. Cowley, PhD, Associate Dean, Graduate School of Social Work, University of Utah, Salt Lake City)*

Published by

The Haworth Social Work Practice Press. 10 Alice Street, Binghamton, NY 13904-1580 USA
The Haworth Social Work Practice Press is an imprint of The Haworth Press, Inc., 10 Alice Street, Binghamton, NY 13904-1580 USA.

Social Work and Divinity has been co-published simultaneously as *Journal of Religion & Spirituality in Social Work: Social Thought*, Volume 24, Numbers 1/2 2005.

Cover design by Kerry E. Mack

Library of Congress Cataloging-in-Publication Data

Social work and divinity/Daniel Lee, Robert O' Gorman, editors.
p.cm.
"Co-published simultaneously as Journal of religion & spirituality in social services, Volume 24, Numbers 1/2 2005"–T.p verso.
Includes bibliographical references and index.
ISBN 0-7890-2756-9 (hard cover: alk. paper)–ISBN 0-7890-2757-7 (soft cover: alk. paper)
1. Pastoral theology–Study and Teaching–Congresses. 2. Social service–Study and teaching–Congresses. 3. Joint academic degree programs–Congresses. I. Lee, Daniel B., 1939- II. O'Gorman, Robert T. (Robert Thomas), 1941-
BV4020.S63 2004
261.8′32–dc22 2004018976

Social Work and Divinity

Daniel Lee
Robert O'Gorman
Guest Editors

Social Work and Divinity has been co-published simultaneously as *Journal of Religion & Spirituality in Social Work: Social Thought*, Volume 24, Numbers 1/2 2005.

The Haworth Social Work Practice Press
The Haworth Pastoral Press
Imprints of The Haworth Press, Inc.

New York • London • Victoria (AU)
www.HaworthPress.com

ALL HAWORTH SOCIAL WORK PRACTICE PRESS
BOOKS AND JOURNALS ARE PRINTED ON
CERTIFIED ACID FREE PAPER.

Indexing, Abstracting & Website/Internet Coverage

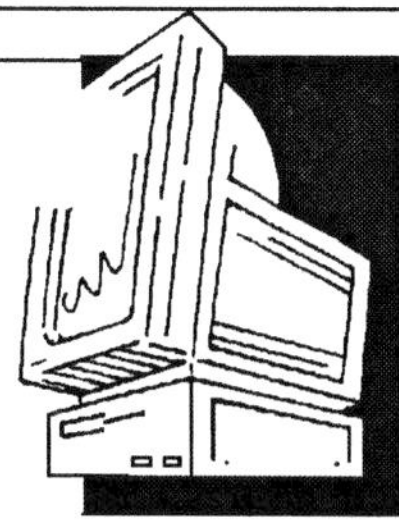

This section provides you with a list of major indexing & abstracting services and other tools for bibliographic access. That is to say, each service began covering this periodical during the year noted in the right column. Most Websites which are listed below have indicated that they will either post, disseminate, compile, archive, cite or alert their own Website users with research-based content from this work. (This list is as current as the copyright date of this publication.)

Abstracting, Website/Indexing Coverage . . . . Year When Coverage Began

- ***Applied Social Sciences Index & Abstracts (ASSIA) (Online: ASSI via Data-Star) (CDRom: ASSIA Plus) <http://www.csa.com>*** **1998**
- ***AURSI African Urban & Regional Science Index. A scholarly & research index which synthesises & compiles all publications on urbanization & regional science in Africa within the world. Published annually*** **2004**
- ***Business Source Corporate: coverage of nearly 3,350 quality magazines and journals; designed to meet the diverse information needs of corporations; EBSCO Publishing <http://www.epnet.com/corporate/bsourcecorp.asp>*** **2004**
- ***CareData: the database supporting social care management and practice <http://www.elsc.org.uk/caredata/caredata.htm>*** **2001**
- ***Catholic Periodical & Literature Index (CPLI), The*** **2001**
- ***CINAHL (Cumulative Index to Nursing & Allied Health Literature), in print, EBSCO, and SilverPlatter, Data-Star, and PaperChase. (Support materials include Subject Heading List, Database Search Guide, and instructional video) <http://www.cinahl.com>*** **2000**

(continued)

- *EAP Abstracts Plus <http://www.eaptechnology.com>* 2003
- *EBSCOhost Electronic Journals Service (EJS); <http://ejournals.ebsco.com>* 2004
- *Family & Society Studies Worldwide <http://www.nisc.com>* 2000
- *FRANCIS. INIST/CNRS <http://www.inist.fr>* 1999
- *Family Index Database <http://www.familyscholar.com>* 2003
- *Google <http://www.google.com>* 2004
- *Google Scholar <http://scholar.google.com>* 2004
- *Guide to Social Science & Religion in Periodical Literature* 1995
- *Haworth Document Delivery Center* 2004
- *IBZ International Bibliography of Periodical Literature <http://www.saur.de>* 1995
- *Index to Jewish Periodicals <http://www.jewishperiodicals.com>* . . . 2001
- *International Review of Biblical Studies. Annual publication of ca. 350 pp. with abstracts of periodical articles & books relevant to biblical studies & related disciplines, especially ancient Near Eastern studies & Egyptology* . . . . *
- *Internationale Bibliographie der geistes- und sozialwissenschaftlichen Zeitschriftenliteratur . . . See IBZ <http://www.saur.de>* 1995
- *Orere Source, The (Pastoral Abstracts)* 1998
- *Pastoral Abstracts (The Journal of Pastoral Care & Counseling) <http://www.jpcp.org>* . . . . *
- *Sage Race Relations Abstracts* 1995
- *Sage Urban Studies Abstracts (SUSA)* 1995
- *Social Services Abstracts <http://www.csa.com>* 1995
- *Social Work Abstracts <http://www.silverplatter.com/catalog/swab.htm>* 1995
- *Sociological Abstracts (SA) <http://www.csa.com>* 1995

(continued)

• *Violence and Abuse Abstracts: A Review of Current Literature on Interpersonal Violence (VAA)* **1995**

***Exact start date to come.**

Special Bibliographic Notes related to special journal issues (separates) and indexing/abstracting:

- indexing/abstracting services in this list will also cover material in any "separate" that is co-published simultaneously with Haworth's special thematic journal issue or DocuSerial. Indexing/abstracting usually covers material at the article/chapter level.
- monographic co-editions are intended for either non-subscribers or libraries which intend to purchase a second copy for their circulating collections.
- monographic co-editions are reported to all jobbers/wholesalers/approval plans. The source journal is listed as the "series" to assist the prevention of duplicate purchasing in the same manner utilized for books-in-series.
- to facilitate user/access services all indexing/abstracting services are encouraged to utilize the co-indexing entry note indicated at the bottom of the first page of each article/chapter/contribution.
- this is intended to assist a library user of any reference tool (whether print, electronic, online, or CD-ROM) to locate the monographic version if the library has purchased this version but not a subscription to the source journal.
- individual articles/chapters in any Haworth publication are also available through the Haworth Document Delivery Service (HDDS).

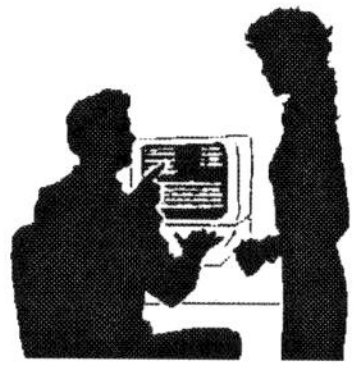

Social Work and Divinity

CONTENTS

ABOUT THE EDITORS

Daniel B. Lee, DSW, is Professor of Social Work and Coordinator for Social Work and Divinity Masters Program, Loyola University Chicago. Dr. Lee joined the Loyola University faculty in 1990 after teaching social work at the Ohio State University for ten years, 1980-1990. He was appointed Associate Dean in 1998. Dr. Lee teaches courses on Religion, Spirituality, and Social Work; Family Diagnosis and Treatment; Ethnicity, Race, and Cultural Diversity; and Clinical Doctoral Seminar. He is founder of the Transcultural Family Institute and also a co-founder and former President of the Global Awareness Society International. His research interests include: Issues of intercultural communication, integration of spirituality and social work, transgenerational family relations, immigrant and relocation stressors, interdisciplinary care and intervention, and marital and family treatment. Dr. Lee is a clinical member of the American Association for Marriage and Family Therapy, 1972-present, and is a licensed marriage and family therapist in the State of Illinois. He currently serves on various boards and in leadership positions of several community, church, and professional organizations. Dr. Lee instituted the First National Symposium on the Integration of Divinity and Social Work Master Programs in 2002. While serving in the U.S. Army Medical Service as a commissioned social work officer for seven years, he lectured at various universities including the University of Hawaii, University of Maryland, Chung Ang University, and Ewha Woman's University. He was also a social worker at the Family Service Agency in Winston-Salem, NC. Dr. Lee was nominated as a Fulbright lecturer, and taught at the Seoul National University in 1995, and Sogang (Jesuit) University in 2002 as a visiting scholar in 1995. His most recent publication includes: *Social Work with Family: Content and Process* (2004), coauthored with Dr. Robert Constable. He currently serves as the president of the Honor Society of International (Phi Beta Delta) Loyola Chapter (2002-04). Dr. Lee is also an ordained United Methodist clergy. Dr. Lee received his graduate social work degrees from the Florida State University (MSW, 1968) and the University of Utah (DSW, 1980).

Robert O'Gorman, PhD, is Professor of Pastoral Studies and Director of Field Communication, the Institute of Pastoral Studies, Loyola University, Chicago. His PhD is from the University of Notre Dame. He came to Loyola in 1989 to direct the newly established MDiv Program. This is a unique MDiv, established as a post-clerical (non-ordination) professional ministerial degree program. Previously he taught at Scarrit Graduate School in Nashville, TN, St. Thomas Seminary in Denver, CO, and the Divinity School of St. Louis University. O'Gorman's research, teaching, and service work has developed in six academic areas: (1) religion and education, (2) theological field education, (3) Hispanic ministry, (4) ministerial identity and theological education, (5) community development and (6) spirituality and the professions. His publications include: *Teaching From a Community Context: The Role of the Field Educator in Theological Education*, a monograph published as a Special Edition of *Theological Education* (2001); *The Complete Idiot's Guide to Understanding Catholicism* (2000); "The Concern for Theological Method in Basic Christian Communities," in *Mapping Christian Education* (1997); *Latin American Theology and Education in Theological Approaches to Christian Education* (1990); *The Church that was a School: Catholic Identity* and *Catholic Education in the United States Since 1790*, (1987); and *The Church in the Education of the Public* (1984). O'Gorman was the recipient of two Association of Theological Schools (ATS) grants, which immersed him in the Hispanic communities of the Southwest and in a community in central Mexico. In 1998 he was a Senior Teaching Scholar at Vanderbilt University. He did research on contextual pedagogies for the 2003 calendar year with a Lilly Foundation grant administered by the Wabash Center for Teaching in Theology and Religion on contextual education in theological schools. During the 1990s he served on the steering committee of the Association of Theological Field Education (ATFE), with the last two years as the Chairperson of this 150 school association of theological field educators. Presently he serves as President of the Religious Education Association of the United States and Canada (REA).

INTRODUCTION

Social Work and Divinity: Directions for Joining These Disciplines in Dual Degree Programs

Daniel Lee
Robert O'Gorman

Toward Building Compassionate Communities: An Integration of Theology and Social Work in Professional Education and Practice was the theme of the First National Symposium on Social Work and Divinity Dual Degree Programs held at Loyola University Chicago, April 19-20, 2002. This ground breaking event was, in part, supported by the grants from the Graduate Studies of Loyola University and the General Board of Higher Education and Ministry Section on Deacons and Diaconal Ministry, the United Methodist Church. The purpose of this symposium was to articulate why such integration of theology and so-

[Haworth co-indexing entry note]: "Social Work and Divinity: Directions for Joining these Disciplines in Dual Degree Programs." Lee, Daniel, and O'Gorman, Robert. Co-published simultaneously in *Journal of Religion & Spirituality in Social Work: Social Thought* (The Haworth Social Work Practice Press, an imprint of The Haworth Press, Inc.) Vol. 24, No. 1/2, 2005, pp. 1-5; and: *Social Work and Divinity* (ed: Daniel Lee, and Robert O'Gorman) The Haworth Social Work Practice Press, an imprint of The Haworth Press, Inc., 2005, pp. 1-5. Single or multiple copies of this article are available for a fee from The Haworth Document Delivery Service [1-800-HAWORTH, 9:00 a.m. - 5:00 p.m. (EST). E-mail address: docdelivery@haworthpress.com].

http://www.haworthpress.com/web/JRSSW

Digital Object Identifier: 10.1300/J377v24n01_01

cial work is so crucial, timely and relevant; and further to examine how these two disciplines can collaborate in building more compassionate communities. The assumption behind this endeavor is that strengthening the scholarly foundations to bridge the knowledge, values and skills these two disciplines bring to professional education and practice will both empower students to serve with commitment and care as well as renew the systems that are purported to serve those in need. Toward this goal, the project initiators and symposium participants joined together to integrate spiritual and social dimensions of care, healing, and services so that these characteristics become more prominent in the areas of teaching, research, training, and practice.

Current trends among academics, mental health practitioners, divinity and social work students, indicate an upsurge of interest in spiritually integrated ways to serve alienated, oppressed, and troubled individuals, families, and small groups. This attempt at integration produces many questions in both theological and practical contexts to meet these challenges.

This symposium raised the following questions for further studies, discussions, and solutions:

- What is the relation between knowing and doing in constructing more relevant interdisciplinary education and practice in light of the call for faith-based social services?
- What is the role of faith and spirituality in education for the dual degree students?
- How do we facilitate collaborative processes between the dual degree programs and field settings to promote more coherent educational experiences for all parties involved?
- How do the dual degree programs relate to institutions in the public sphere and the churches?
- How do students form a dual professional identity; and what contributes to a healthy level of integration throughout their developmental phases of identity formation and role acquisition?
- Does a distinction in the terms: *religion, faith, spirituality, divinity,* and *theology* lead social work to a more comprehensive, and yet differential approach, in serving the client systems?
- What does it take for dual degree students and practitioners to engage more effectively in building globally holistic and culturally resourceful approaches to the people who need advocacy, mediation and healing?

In addition to examining the current status of the divinity and social work dual degree programs, this symposium aimed at the development of successive contributions expanding the scope of interests and expertise in a *theology of social work* for dual degree programs.

Papers from this symposium are organized around nine sub themes followed by a conclusion. The first sub theme, "Ecological, Societal Spiritual Regeneration: A Cosmic Foundation for Integration," is authored by Edward "Joe" Holland, PhD, who is Professor of Philosophy and Religion at St. Thomas University, and President of Pax Romana USA, a Catholic Movement for Intellectual & Cultural Affairs. Holland explores the nature of postmodern planetary civilization, which we are only beginning to enter. In his paper, he addresses the need for what might be called ecological, societal, and spiritual regeneration of life across the planet, in the wake of the breakdown of modern culture. Katherine Tyson, MDiv, PhD, Professor of Social Work, Loyola University Chicago underscores Holland's vision of a postmodern return to technologically-empowered communities, and advances her position describing the relevance of a revolutionary psychology of the human condition, *intrapsychic humanism,* as progress towards a just social order. She maintains developmental care giving relationships are powerful means for establishing just communities and bringing about the satisfaction of each individual's quest for a personally meaningful life.

The second sub theme, "Curricular Integration: Common and Distinctive Elements" authored by Homer Ashby, PhD, Professor of Theology at McCormick Theological Seminary, Chicago stresses that the divinity and social work curriculum in dual degree programs should clarify for students the distinctiveness and the common elements of their mutual commitment to work toward the health and wholeness of individuals and communities. He explores those common elements and distinctive features, and even recommends that the name of such programs be changed from dual degree programs to joint degree programs.

In the third sub theme, "Integration of Religious and Spiritual Beliefs in a Social Work Course," Professor Terry Northcut, PhD, Loyola University Chicago, discusses the role of religion and spirituality in clinical social work as one of the most visible means to meet the needs of clients and to examine both our and our clients' religious and spiritual beliefs. She cautions against too much formative curriculum development as a solution to the ambiguities inherent in dual degree programs.

The fourth sub theme, "Professional Identity Formation of Dual Degree Students," Robert O'Gorman, Professor of Pastoral Studies at Loyola Chicago, poses an important question of dual identity for dual degree students who are often left alone without critical examinations of their professional dual identity in their formation processes. In particular, O'Gorman explores reflections on the experiences of dual degree students in the context of the Clinical Pastoral Education and students' experiences negotiating this requirement.

Margaret Ann Crain, PhD, from Garrett-Evangelical Theological Seminary, Chicago, describes the new order of deacon within the United Methodist Church in her paper (sub-theme 5) entitled: "The Diaconate as Dual-Skilled Ministry: A Proposal in Support of Dual Degree Programs for Formation" Crain argues that the complexities of understanding systems that lead to oppression and the call to do justice, love and mercy require creative approaches such as dual degree programs in divinity and social work. She also notes the important role of the ecclesiastical bodies that supervise programs of formation and education in supporting students with money, time and encouragement.

Most Reverend Edwin M. Conway, MDiv, MSW, DD, Auxiliary Bishop of the Catholic Archdiocese of Chicago, authors sub-theme 6, "Collaborative Responses to the Demands of Emerging Human Needs: The Role of Faith and Spirituality in Education for Social Work." Bishop Conway focuses on the integration of faith and social work from a Catholic point of view. By critically reflecting on historical discourse between the fields of social work and religion, he delineates many aspects of natural integration between spirituality and social work. He offers practical suggestions to stimulate more profound thinking on the development of the dual degree program.

Edward Canda, PhD, Professor of Social Work at University of Kansas offers insights, examples and suggestions for "Integrating Religion and Social Work in Dual Degree Programs" (sub-theme 7). By elaborating his own personal journey in trying to find ways to connect religious studies, pastoral counseling, and social work, Canda describes beneficial challenges from religion to social work and from social work to religion. Several practical suggestions are provided for designing integrated religion and social work dual degree programs.

"On Social Work Environment: The Locus of Integration" (sub theme 8), Ram Cnaan, PhD, Professor of Social Work at University of Pennsylvania introduces a course entitled: *Practicing and Managing Social Work in Religious Context*. Noting the emergence of religion as a social force in America, Cnaan prepares his students working in and with faith-based organizations. He covers the rationale for the course, the process in building the curriculum, the experience with his teaching, and current student evaluations. He discusses aspects of extending the school's public discourse to include religion and enhancing relationships with local theological schools.

Holly Nelson-Becker, PhD, University of Kansas at Lawrence, examines the perceived importance and professional integration of both religion and spirituality in clinical practice by two groups of master's level of social work graduates, one having a second master's degree in religion/divinity in her empirical study: "Does a Dual Degree Make a Difference in Social Work: An Empirical Study" (Sub theme 9). Her findings indicate that both groups endorse the value of including a spiritual dimension in holistic treatment of clients and the need for addressing religious and spiritual issues in professional social work training. Both groups, however, struggle to integrate religion and spirituality in professional practice. Implications for social work include the benefits of dialoguing with dual degree social work colleagues who can contribute to our understanding of religion and spirituality in a professional context.

In conclusion, Daniel Lee, DSW, Professor of Social Work at Loyola University Chicago, who organized the symposium, reflects upon the current trends in emerging dual degree programs between divinity and social work schools in the United States and the importance of conversing between the two professions to expand the integrated curriculum developments and to network among the dual degree graduates. He proposes that a more holistic approach be employed in strengthening dual degree programs both conceptually and practically to advance our understanding of human nature that includes the dimension of spirituality and the complexity of social issues. Several recommendations and suggestions are provided toward building more compassionate communities through the means of equipping our students and practitioners with integrated values, knowledge and skills in professional practices.

The Regeneration of Ecological, Societal, and Spiritual Life: The Holistic Postmodern Mission of Humanity in the Newly Emerging Planetary Civilization

Joe Holland

SUMMARY. This paper proposes that the Electronic Revolution has triggered the emergence of a fourth era in human cultural-technological

---

Edward "Joe" Holland, PhD, is Professor of Philosophy and Religion at St. Thomas University. A philosopher and theologian specializing in the relationship between religion and society, he holds a PhD from the University of Chicago and was a Fulbright Scholar at the Universidad Católica in Santiago, Chile. He is Senior Scholar with the International Consortium on Religion and Ecology in Washington, DC, a member of the Associate Faculty of New York Theological Seminary in New York City, Adjunct Professor at Drew University's School of Theology in Madison, NJ, and State Coordinator of the Florida Council of Catholic Scholarship. In addition, he is President of the United States Federation of Pax Romana-International Catholic Movement for Intellectual and Cultural Affairs.

Address correspondence to: Joe Holland, St. Thomas University, Miami, FL, (E-mail: JoeHolland@aol.com).

Printed with permission.

[Haworth co-indexing entry note]: "The Regeneration of Ecological, Societal, and Spiritual Life: The Holistic Postmodern Mission of Humanity in the Newly Emerging Planetary Civilization." Holland, Joe. Co-published simultaneously in *Journal of Religion & Spirituality in Social Work: Social Thought* (The Haworth Social Work Practice Press, an imprint of The Haworth Press, Inc.) Vol. 24, No. 1/2, 2005, pp. 7-25; and: *Social Work and Divinity* (ed: Daniel Lee, and Robert O'Gorman) The Haworth Social Work Practice Press, an imprint of The Haworth Press, Inc., 2005, pp. 7-25. Single or multiple copies of this article are available for a fee from The Haworth Document Delivery Service [1-800-HAWORTH, 9:00 a.m. - 5:00 p.m. (EST). E-mail address: docdelivery@haworthpress.com].

http://www.haworthpress.com/web/JRSSW
Digital Object Identifier: 10.1300/J377v24n01_02

evolution, namely a (multicultural) postmodern planetary civilization. This new era builds on the prior eras: (1) the primal-tribal era of speech; (2) the classical-imperial-city-state era of writing; and (3) the modern nation-state era of mechanical printing. In this new global era, human society is seen as called to ground its cultural-spiritual structures in the "creative communion of life," its political-governmental structures in "local-global networks," and its techno-economic structures in micro-technologies, micro-finance, and micro-enterprises, all of which would be ecological in character. Within this new historical context, professionals in religion and social work are called to form fresh generations of young leaders through an alternative educational system that would point toward a postmodern movement of ecological, social, and spiritual regeneration linked to new monastic-like centers of the fresh vision. *[Article copies available for a fee from The Haworth Document Delivery Service: 1-800-HAWORTH. E-mail address: <docdelivery@haworthpress.com> Website: <http://www.HaworthPress.com>*

KEYWORDS. Ecology, society, spirituality, modern, postmodern, civilization, electronics, culture, evolution

In this paper, I would like to explore the nature of the new postmodern planetary civilization which we are only beginning to enter, and in particular to address the need for what might be called the ecological, societal, and spiritual regeneration of life across the planet, in the wake of the breakdown of modern culture.

MODERN BREAKDOWN AND POSTMODERN BREAKTHROUGH

The 500 year cycle of modern civilization is now coming to an end. This modern world was a creation of the modern European male bourgeoisie. Like all civilizations, it has given us rich and abiding gifts–for example, a cherishing of individual human rights, the creation of popular democracy, an explosion of technological creativity, and an expansion of the *devotio moderna's* psychologically oriented spirituality of interiority. We need always be grateful for these rich gifts, and make sure that we preserve and even expand them for future generations.

Modernity's Foundational Evils

But, as with all civilizations, the modern world also contained foundational evils. We might recall first the racial and class exploitations that enabled the modern European bourgeoisie to rise to power. These exploitations included: seizing the lands and resources of the native peoples of the Americas while inflicting on many of their peoples a near genocide; enslaving or killing in attempted enslavement nearly 50 million African youth; driving much of the Western European peasantry off the lands which they had worked in common from time immemorial, and then exploiting them as the proletariat of early industrial capitalism; and unleashing a new and brutal wave of industrial colonialism on Africa and Asia.

In another foundational evil, modern Eurocentric culture promoted a mechanistic hyper-masculine of paradigm of science and technology. Promoted by the modern secular university system and applied to all major institutions, this paradigm progressively marginalized women's historically essential contributions to socio-economic life. Since the birth of human culture, women's ways had provided the grounding webs and cycles for the human community and for humanity's wider community with nature. But modernity suppressed these ancient feminine communal ways and instead gradually tried to restructure all of human experience, beginning with economic experience around the masculine way of competition. This masculine way, also an essential component of social life, was developed over tens of thousands of years mostly in warfare against enemies and in long-distance trading of exotic commodities.

The imbalanced maximization of the masculine way has resulted today is a colossal masculine global market culture centered both in a gargantuan and dangerous military-industrial complex and in a frenetic and sacrilegious consumerist cult of what Karl Marx called the "commodity fetish." The whole process is now wrecking vast ecological, societal, and spiritual devastation across the planet.

> So, at the start of the 21st century and of the third millennium of Christianity, we stand amidst the final and life-threatening climax of the 500-year-old modern attempt to reshape all global community, both societal and ecological, in the Eurocentric bourgeois hyper-masculine image. Now we gaze out upon the environmental, familial, and ecclesial devastation of late modern culture.

Unexpectedly we discover, as has been proclaimed recently by so many analysts, that the modern way of life is not sustainable. It is not sustainable ecologically. It is not sustainable societally. And it is not sustainable ecclesially. So quite suddenly in both society and religion, we find ourselves suffering the harsh and confusing pain of the terminal crisis of modernity.

Modern Print and Postmodern Electronics

The modern world arose primarily because the European print revolution gave the expanding bourgeois classes a powerful communications instrument by which to challenge the societal hegemony of the traditional Catholic aristocracy. The Catholic aristocracy had maintained its 5,000 plus years of control by the use of handwriting in an elite language, Latin in the European case. In the classical world the ancient egalitarian tribes, whom the aristocratic warriors had conquered remained confined to the limited pre-classical medium of speech; the tribal peoples were illiterate and so powerless to gain access to the controlling aristocratic information system. Only the aristocracy, or alternately the clerical class of priests and monks, could afford expensive tutors for their youth. Equally expensive handwritten texts provided the aristocracy with both imperial standardization of information and mystical legitimization for their class "superiority."

But with the 15th century introduction of mechanical printing into Europe, relatively cheap publications suddenly brought literacy to the expanding middle classes. Quickly, print provided a public medium for exposing the great injustice and repression that had grounded and sustained the ancient aristocratic system. Print was thus a revolutionary medium, and its communicative power stood behind all the major bourgeois revolutions–the Protestant Reformation, the Scientific Revolution, the Enlightenment, the French and American democratic revolutions, and finally the Industrial Revolution. By contrast, central to the aristocracy's failed attempt at counter-revolution was the censorship and suppression of subversive printed information.

Today modern print-based bourgeois hegemony is itself being undermined by the postmodern electronic revolution. In the short run, the electronic revolution's creation of global networks of transportation, communication, and information has enabled the modern capitalist enterprise to mushroom from its past form as the national managerial oligopoly to its new shape as the transnational strategic conglomerate. This is the phenomenon we know as "globalization."

But in the long run, I propose, the electronic revolution will undermine the entire modern bourgeois project. For example, I propose that the electronic revolution, because its micro-scale is inherently decentralizing, offers the possibility of returning re-rooting socio-economic life in the local community and even in the familial household. Narrating a recent incident may illustrate this decentralizing feature.

Recently Xabier Gorostiaga, formerly the President of the Jesuit-sponsored University in Nicaragua, told me that, thanks to the acquisition of 500 inexpensive old-generation computers distributed by his university to remote rural villages, the teenage daughters of poor and illiterate Nicaraguan peasants are now tracking through the Internet the daily fluctuations of the world-market price of corn. And thanks to constant email communications with their new electronic girl friends across rural Nicaragua, these teenagers have formed a cooperative marketing process that bypasses traditional regional brokers and determines the best timing for direct marketing. As a result, the peasants have doubled the sale-price of their harvest.

While the preceding example is the realm of primary production, the same is true in the realm of finance. As is now well know from the many stories of replications of the famous Grameen Bank. Communities of poor women, when provided with very small loans, prove to have better rates of return than the US "Fortune 500" top companies. And, in contrast to the more masculine style of competitive long-distance trading favored by modern capitalist enterprises, women tend to use capital to build up the local economic community, beginning with their own extended families. Processing, tracking, and multiplying such small loans are greatly facilitated by computers.

It is perhaps appropriate to recall here that "the market," a social invention tens of thousands of years older than capitalism, was originally created by and for millennia under the control of local women, as still can be seen in the traditional *mercados* (markets) of the native peoples of Latin America.

A Fourth Era in Human Evolution

The postmodern electronic revolution needs to be contextualized within the general story of the historical evolution of human culture thus far, and particularly from a Western perspective since, for better or worse, Western culture has emerged as hegemonic planetary influence at the start of the postmodern era (Holland, 1992).[1]

First, perhaps some 40,000 years ago, ago humanity entered its primal era of human culture. This era saw the emergence of decentralized and egalitarian tribal communities based on the communications medium of speech. These communities were still immersed in the "feminine" webs and cycles of nature, and centered their culture life in what has been at least historically women's cyclical and connecting style. Further, these communities expressed themselves in a predominately "feminine" integration of science and religion, oriented especially to the maternal face of God usually understood as an Earth-mother goddess (Holy Bible, Genesis, 1:27).[2]

Second, perhaps some 5,000 years ago, aristocratic classical civilizations began to emerge across the planet. These were crudely centralized imperial systems of elite city-based control. Their aristocratic "higher" cultures, based on stone and metal construction, reigned above the "lower" and organic peasant systems surviving from the primal era. The communications medium of these classical empires was handwriting, produced in an elite language. These empires, in their elite spheres, imposed a linear and separating phallic style as their expression of so-called higher culture. In so doing, they established a new masculine paradigm integrating science and religion, and placed it hierarchically above the ancient feminine wisdom, which still continued among subservient peasants. At the elite level, these empires looked more to the paternal face of God, usually understood as a sky-father, while the so-called lower peasant class continued to be drawn more to the feminine Earth-mother image of the divine. While the paternal face of God has its own legitimacy, its aristocratic imperial expression severely distorted that authenticity. The preaching and deeds of Jesus brought us back to a more authentic divine *abba* (Holy Bible, Mark, 9:35).[3]

Third, some 500 years ago, the European bourgeoisie set out to recreate the whole world in its own image, and thus launched the modern form of human civilization. As mentioned, this form's leading means of communications has been print. The modern world emerged as a Eurocentric cluster of competitively nationalistic societies, in which the urban bourgeoisie came to exercise control covertly and indirectly through the public and private bureaucracies of liberal government and liberal business. The modern era has represented a dramatic intensification of the patriarchal drive that began with the origins of classical civilization.

In contrast to classicism, modernity dualistically placed religion in a separate "feminine" sphere of interiorized psychological spiritualities, while it placed science in a separate "masculine" sphere of exteriorized mechanistic technologies. Nonetheless, the institutional expressions of both religion and science remained under firm bourgeois male control. In this process, the masculine scientific spirit lost its spiritual roots, while expanding its embodiment in business and the military as a secularized and competitive male mystique of phallic "mission" guided by a managerial ethos. Meanwhile the feminine religious spirit lost its technological embodiment, while having its spiritual roots re-tailored in a modern cult of domesticity. This was expressed in home as a center of consumerism, pietistic religion, and the "helping professions," with all symbolized as a caring yet privatized mystique of womb-like "community" guided by a therapeutic ethos (Bellah, 1966).[4]

In the late modern crisis at the institutional level, the two cultural energies of science and religion have increasingly become structured in their bourgeois form as a symbolically masculine violent addiction and a self-negating symbolically feminine codependency. The mutually destructive result is a threatening late modern "culture of death," to use the phrasing of Pope John Paul II. I like to speak of a mutually dysfunctional "dance of death" between bourgeois science and technology on one side, and bourgeois religion and spirituality on the other. Breaking out of this dance of death requires undertaking a healing journey into a holistic postmodern vision.

The inevitability of the electronic era does not mean that the transition to the fourth or *postmodern* era of human civilization will be simple or smooth. In all past history, the emergence of a new long-term cultural cycle has always meant violent social upheaval. Already across the planet we are seeing an explosion of both low-intensity and high-intensity local wars. In the future there may be many more such wars, particularly civil wars. To help reduce this violence of the transition, I will now propose a healing and holistic vision of postmodern social strategy.

FOUR ERAS OF WESTERN CULTURAL EVOLUTION

These may be called "stages" but really are concentric circles. Also, the human story begins in Africa, has now become planetary, yet retains its African foundation.

STAGE	SOCIETY	COMMUNICATIONS	SPIRITUALITY	SEXUAL SYMBOL
Primal 40,000 bce	Tribe Organic Metaphor	Speech Women's Technologies (Instrumental Male)	Immanence Women's Spiritualities (Instrumental Male)	Earth Mother Nature Religions (Womb-like circle)
Classical 5,000 bce	Empire Hierarchical Metaphor	Writing Men's Technologies (Above Women)	Transcendence Men's Spiritualities (Above Women)	Sky Father Priestly Religion (Phallic Line)
Modern 1,500 ce	Nation Mechanistic Metaphor	Print Secularization of Men's Technologies (Mission/Product)	Interiority Privatization of Women's Spiritualities (Community/ Process)	Sibling Rivalry Pietistic Religion (vs. Mechanistic Science)
Post-Planet modern 2,000 ce	Electronics Artistic Metaphor	Co-Creativity Female/Male Technological Synthesis	Fertile Embrace Female/Male Spiritual Synthesis	Ecological Religion (Bipolar Regeneration)

TOWARD A HOLISTIC POSTMODERN VISION

As we have seen, the primal speech revolution enabled small familial bands to be woven into larger organic-immanent tribal communities. The classical handwriting revolution gave the aristocratic elites of some city-states the standardized information records necessary to sustain hierarchical-transcendent imperial domination over vast numbers of tribal groups. The modern print revolution enabled the emerging bourgeoisie to break-up the Western imperial system into vernacular nation-states, and then to spread the liberal ideology of mechanistic capitalism to the entire world-community.

Now because of the electronic revolution, and under the leadership of both local and global information elites, the autonomous sovereignty of national systems may begin to yield to an ecological-artistic global/local symbiosis embracing and integrating the entire planet. In this projected postmodern breakthrough, the innovative mode of communications becomes electronic and the societal scale becomes planetary. But the planetary scale simultaneously favors decentralized rooting in local communities, thus giving us a local/global structural paradigm.

Culture and Spirituality: The Creative Communion of Life

The spirituality of this new stage flows from an artistic root metaphor (in contrast to modernity's mechanistic metaphor or classicism's hierarchical root-metaphor), and is centered in the energy-flow of the creative communion of ecological, human, and divine life. This energy-flow is seen as sexually in a partnership of the feminine and masculine symbols, and humanly expressed especially in the sacred tasks of family, work, and citizenship (Holland, 1992).[5]

The deepest level of this postmodern transition is the dawning ecological consciousness. Thomas Berry has called this a new era in the Earth process itself–the shift from the Cenozoic to the Ecozoic Age. The Cenozoic refers to the past 67 million years when life spontaneously exploded after the extinction of the dinosaurs. The Ecozoic is the new era wherein all evolutionary geological and biological processes are increasingly intertwined with human technological intervention, and human consciousness comes to understand itself as part of Earth's own unfolding.

As this postmodern consciousness emerges, the foundational ethical question becomes whether the vastly expanded human power of technological intervention into natural and social ecology will enhance or diminish the planetary community of life (Berry & Swimme, 1988).[6] This ethical question is at the heart of the juncture between the modern breakdown and the postmodern breakthrough. By competing revisions of the liberal ideology, late modern neoconservatives and late modern neoprogressives are attempting to defend the modern cultural project from fundamental breakdown. Yet as the ecological and social crises intensify, the modern project becomes increasing dysfunctional, due to the increasing loss of creative communion with the webs and cycles (space and time) of natural and social ecology, as well as with the ecological and social dimension of the religious Mystery.

The positive side of the postmodern cultural breakthrough may now be seen only seminally in decentralized, flexible, creative, local-global networks functioning across a range of collective identities more complex than class–for example, gender, age, ecology, race, ethnicity, etc. Yet the class factor by no means disappears. Rather it is itself reshaped and re-expressed across this diffused community of decentralized symbolic movements.[7]

In the late modern breakdown and postmodern breakthrough, the primary social struggle becomes less immediately over political-economic power and more profoundly over cultural-spiritual meaning, though with powerful political-economic implications. Culture and its deeper root in spirituality then become the central spheres of the transition.

In this struggle for the emergence of a regenerative postmodern cultural vision, the ecosystem itself becomes the model for our technologies and a source of our spiritualities. This perspective represents a shift from the socially centered or anthropocentric consciousness of the receding modern culture to the ecologically centered or biocentric consciousness of the emerging postmodern culture (Toffler, 1992).[8] To repeat, this breakthrough would no longer be based on the modern anthropocentric assumptions of the liberal ideology's autonomous human freedom and progress, but rather on an entirely fresh postmodern biocentric ecological vision of the creative communion of ecological, human, and divine life. The question then arises, in what political policies would such a vision be embodied?

Reigning policies linked to reactionary defense of late modern civilization support the centralization of the transnational conglomerates, particularly fossil-fuel based energy companies, with all the repressive and marginalizing state policies that implies. However, alternative policies seeking postmodern regeneration would support a decentralization of social life, particularly in energy (for example, solar power), working patterns, and communications. Increasingly this alternative scenario is described as "sustainable communities" (Catholic Committee of Appalachia, 1995).[9] Let us imagine what such bioregional, yet globally networked, sustainable communities might look like.

Politics and Government: Local-Global Networks

The electronic revolution leads to the primacy of globally connected networks of holistic local communities artistically adapted to the ecologies of their particular bioregions, and re-rooted in the familial household, with a diminished role for the nation-state. These local communities would contain sophisticated electronic information systems and craft-based electronic production systems, all linked to global networks of communication and transportation (Toffler, 1992).[10] In this process, the presently growing role of mega-cities, begun seminally in the classical imperial stage and expanded dramatically throughout the modern industrial age, would recede.

This would mark a return to the primacy of the local village, which was the predominant shape of social organization for tens of thousands of years prior to classicism and modernity, and still is in many areas of the planet. Yet villages would be networked into a global family through electronic grids of communication and transportation. The ancient village system would be recreated and enhanced as part of a planetary electronic network. Cities would remain, but they would be returned to a smaller scale than that of the expanding mega-cities of today (Toffler, 1992).[11]

Also, because of easy and inexpensive computerized access to sophisticated information, ordinary households and communities of households will probably recapture control over major social functions. Following print-based modernization, they lost this control to university-trained, specialized professionals. Examples include health-care, law, education, and religion. With advanced forms of data systems, the postmodern household will be able to access rich information in all these professional areas, to employ it with new self-help models, and to do so with low-cost, user-friendly instruments similar to contemporary inexpensive televisions, telephones, and video-games. Specially trained professionals in distinct institutional areas will remain important, but their main task will be to provide households and communities with the systematized information and with procedural guidance for its retrieval and application.[12]

At the same time, the role of the nation-state will diminish not only internally in its centralizing bureaucracy but also externally in its political sovereignty, and the role of regional and global political institutions will increase. It is interesting to recall that in international law the nation-state only became a sovereign jurisdiction only in 1648, with the Peace of Westphalia following the European religious-military conflicts known as the Thirty Years War. Prior to that time, political authority had been largely divided between supra-national imperial hierarchies and local aristocratic leadership. Now, with growing planetary consciousness, it becomes clear that nation-states can no longer reign sovereign in the face of growing regional and planetary social and ecological crises. Regional and planetary authorities will develop significant military and police structures, as well as taxing power. How all this is to be accomplished, while retaining and even deepening a commitment to participatory democracy, is a major political question for the postmodern period (Falk & Mendlovitz, 1966).[13]

The model of political organizing is also shifting. The second phase of industrial capitalism precipitated the creation of mass political parties and other mass social organizations, all serviced by relatively anonymous elites staffing centralized national bureaucracies and aimed at influencing the central political apparatus of the nation-state through mass force. By contrast, the development of electronic technologies has shifted the organizational initiative from centrally managed bureaucracies to decentralized networks of creative chaos (Prigogine & Stengers, 1984).[14]

As this new postmodern model of politics emerges, we logically experience an intensifying crisis of the mass-industrial style of modern bureaucratic political parties, modern bureaucratic trade unions, modern bureaucratic religious institutions, etc. Increasingly occupying the space once held by these bureaucratic structures are new chaotic and pluralistic networks. It is these chaotic and pluralistic networks that often represent the bearers of the new culture. As mentioned earlier, the cultural struggle carried by these movements becomes central (Gomez de Souza, 1992).[15]

The new information power of electronic networks provides a richer and more diverse flow of information to the grass-roots, making possible much more intense, though more chaotic models of political organization and participation. At the moment these networks appear spontaneous and unstable, but as postmodern communities become themselves become more rooted, these networks will mature into important carriers of decentralized organization and participation.

The transition to a decentralized but networked communitarian village-household model may grow initially out of the economic marginalization of the underclass. As neither private nor public institutions will provide employment or adequate compensatory services for the growing global underclass, there could well be a long period of social unrest and upheaval, including extensive class and regional violence. In the midst of such violence, however, hopefully regenerative local communities will begin to gather defensively around the newly decentralized electronic tools, much as the ancient Benedictine monasteries originally sprung up in response to the turmoil of early feudalism precipitated by the fall of the Roman Empire.

Labor unions, community organizations, political parties, and religious bodies might begin to lead movements of the marginalized urban poor to projects of rural re-colonization, supported by postmodern electronic technologies. Such movements could learn from the more ancient village model still in place in many areas of the world, or even from certain contemporary Western religious movements that deliberately resisted the path of liberal modernization, for example the Hutterites, the Amish, and the Mennonites, all of whom have maintained sustainable communities (Stephenson, 1991).[16]

Technology and Economics: Micro-Technology, Micro-Finance, and Micro-Enterprise

These postmodern local communities with their productive households will include self-reliant bases of organic agriculture, perhaps more on a model of small-scale intensive horticulture, rather on the modern industrial model of large-scale mechanistic agriculture (so heavily dependent on dangerous petrochemical inputs). Food production, like all postmodern technological processes, will become artistically and ecologically specific to local bioregions, and will draw on the genetic richness of local plant life, in contrast to the standardized monocultures of transnational agribusiness (so ecologically vulnerable because of their lack of genetic diversity). In addition, food production will move away from intense commercial refinement and packaging, drop down lower on the food chain, and reflect a cheaper, healthier, and more ecological diet (Brown, 1981).[17]

The energy systems for these local communities will be largely based on renewable, non-polluting sources. Key will be solar energy and biomass, giving greater economic strength to the tropical and semi-tropical regions of the planet, which are often areas inhabited by economically poorer and darker-skinned peoples. Where more intense and mobile applications were required, energy might be provided by hydrogen gas, or perhaps one day on a large scale by clean nuclear fusion. The overall use of energy will be marked by much higher levels of efficiency, due to high priority given to conservation and to natural heating and cooling techniques (Brown, 1991).[18]

In addition, we are now on the verge of an explosion of desktop manufacturing, in which relatively inexpensive computers will be connected to relatively inexpensive industrial devices. Perhaps the first major development will be the linking of the microcomputer with a small sewing machine. When this happens, most of the world's garment industry will probably leave the factory and return to the home, presumably under the control of women. And, as Alvin Toffler predicted in *The Third Wave* (1988), eventually the same movement will occur in the many industries that provide basic manufacturing products.

Further, as both solar energy collectors and satellite dishes become smaller and less expensive, such developments will spread quickly over even remote areas of the planet. In the centralized modern age, national industrial "development" required massive investments in a heavy infrastructure of power plants, of railways, roads and bridges, and of cable systems for electricity and telephone. In the decentralized postmodern age, so-called "under-developed" regions will leapfrog over the national industrial era and go directly to the technologically light and locally based electronic mode of production, with easy access global interaction.

For example, in Miami, Florida where I teach, many of the students come from small "underdeveloped" Caribbean islands. Already the people of many of those small islands are bypassing traditional landline telephone systems and going straight to cellular phones. Similarly many of these same students go on to work in very small family-based regional trading enterprises. The fax machine, electronic mail, and the cell phone have given these micro-enterprises the same communicative power as the largest transnational conglomerates. In addition, corporate bureaucracies do not encumber these micro-enterprises.

Thus, thanks to the newly emerging electronic age, we will probably eventually see the end of much of most of the modern factory system (apart from large complex products), undermined by a massive return on a global scale to home or village based production in the artisan-craft model, but now in electronically enhanced form. The combination of micro-technologies with micro-finance will mean a global explosion of micro-enterprise.

In all of this, the role of technology will not be reduced, as if technology itself were the problem; rather technology will be artistically transformed. We will rediscover that technology is not some unidirectional monolithic imperative (locked into the modern idea of mechanistic "progress"). Rather it covers a wide range of artistic paths and styles, among which communities may create according to their own bioregional and cultural imagination. The tendency called "appropriate technology" represents a movement in this direction (McRobie, 1981).[19]

I believe leaders of many transnational conglomerates already understand the threatening implications of this decentralizing postmodern process, for they are increasingly concentrating their strategies on the control of patents and information. With all of these systemic economic changes, the role of multinational conglomerates would be reduced, but not eliminated. These organizations would probably provide many of the global networks of communication, transportation, and information, as well as manufactured products that required a scale larger than local electronic craft production.

The question might then be asked whether or not this postmodern global-local model would still be called capitalism. If by capitalism one means a strong place for the principles of commercial trading and private property, then the answer would be yes. But this, I propose, is a superficial understanding of capitalism since, as noted earlier, such practices are far more ancient than capitalism itself.

There will be a profound postmodern shift away from the modern liberal concept of the autonomy of capital from nature and humanity. Thus, if by capitalism one means the principle of the priority of capital over labor and over Earth, then the society would probably no longer be understood as capitalist, and some other name for the economic system would seem more appropriate. But whatever the name, in the new model the organization of capital would be seen as embedded within and accountable to the ecological, social, and spiritual communities from which it arises. Capital would be accountable to labor, both would be accountable to Earth, and all would be seen as flowing from creative communion with the religious Mystery.

Though all of this sounds optimistic, the political transition to this global-local electronic political model could bring, as already suggested, turbulent and bloody local wars, as was the case with the rise of the earlier classical imperial or modern national eras. As we have already seen with the breakup of the Soviet imperial state, and more recently with the threatening presence of violent Muslim extremists, the resulting vacuum gives rise to ancient demons of ethnic and cultural hatred. In addition, the new technology makes more feasible the threat of supra-national terrorist movements, rooted in local communities which often bypass or rebel against national political elites. In this context, therefore, the need for increasing socially and religiously inspired "dialogue among civilizations," for democratically guided regional and global institutions of political order, and even for global and regional police and military structures, as well as for regional and global taxing powers, becomes paramount.

IMPLICATIONS FOR RELIGION AND SOCIAL WORK

Before concluding, it may be helpful to offer a few brief reflections on the postmodern transition may mean for the two fields of religion and social work, and particularly for their institutional contexts.

First, we need to realize that, since we stand in the middle of a vast cultural transformation, all present institutional structures, formed historically in response to the functioning of modern culture, are inevitably showing themselves, simply because of historical inertial, to be profoundly dysfunctional before the challenges of the postmodern local/global cultural context. These institutions include not only economic and political structures, but also religion, education, and social work. It will be some time before these institutions are adequately transformed in a way that responds creatively and critically to the new context.

Thus, even while we work for and await that large institutional transformation, it becomes important to create small pioneering alternatives in dialogue with the wider institutional structures. For this to happen, it will be necessary to create alternative educational tracks, grounded in the new cultural vision, and to form a fresh generation of young leaders for these institutions, and especially to form young leaders coming especially from poor communities across the Earth. The new networks of electronic communications could prove resourceful here.

Second, to help create and sustain these pioneering alternatives, it will be necessary to create an infrastructure of professionals devoted to create the new institutional paths for all professions. Such an infrastructure might be called a postmodern global "monastic" movement of regeneration. After the fall of the Roman Empire, the European monastic movement created the foundation for a new and eventually modern civilization. Today small local communities of devoted professionals, who would be committed to the new vision and who would be network globally, could play a similar role in the postmodern context. Most important, such a movement would have to be centered in rural re-colonization, and simultaneously in land reform across the planet.

Third, such professionals forming communities of regeneration would need to be grounded in a regenerative postmodern spirituality, which elsewhere I have described as an ecologically grounded spirituality of creative communion, capable of supporting the regeneration of ecological, societal, and spiritual life both locally and on a planetary scale (Holland, 1989).[20]

CONCLUSION

In conclusion, if my analysis is correct, we are seeing the emergence of a fresh postmodern planetary stage in the journey of human development, entailing a profound transformation of human structures and consciousness. In that transformation, the great postmodern mission for all humanity, including its societal and religious institutions, becomes the planetary regeneration of ecological, societal, and spiritual life.

In that mission, we hear the call for holistic strategies that will bring to consciousness the deep connections with always existed between religion and society–as a challenge to both the modern bourgeois secularization and society and the modern bourgeois privatization of religion. In this process, academic programs that link the study of religion and the study of society can play a major role in supporting both compassionate and sustainable communities as the leading edge of the new civilization.

NOTES

1. This analysis of humanity's cultural evolution is based on my monograph, *The Postmodern Electronic Era: Myth, Sexual Symbol, and Technological Function* (Washington DC: The Warwick Institute, 1992).

2. Genesis 1:27 tells us that there are two incomplete images of God, one masculine and one feminine, which together make the full image of God: "God created the Earth-creature (Adam) in his image; in the divine image he created them; male and female he created him."

3. While Jesus resorted the authentic masculine vision of the paternal divine, he nonetheless forbid his disciples to appropriate it for themselves–so great was the masculine temptation of religious infection by the repressive aristocratic paradigm. See, for example, Mark 9:35, 10:15, 12:38-40; Matthew 20:25-28, 23:8-10.

4. On the managerial ethos and therapeutic ethos, which correspond respectively to the instrument and expressive sides of the liberal ideology, see Robert Bellah et al., *Habits of the Heart: Individualism and Commitment in American Life* (University of California Press, 1966).

5. Holland, "The Postmodern Electronic Era," pp. 9-12.

6. See Berry and Swimme, *The Universe Story: From the Primordial Flaring Forth to the Ecozoic Era–a Celebration of the Unfolding of the Cosmos* (San Francisco: Harper, 1994), pp. 240-261.

7. For rich statements of this perspective, see Charlene Spretnak, *The Spiritual Dimension of Green Politics* (Santa Fe, New Mexico: Bear & Co., 1986); Berry & Swimme, *Universe Story*; Berry, *Dream of the Earth* (San Francisco: Sierra Club, 1988); Rupert Sheldrake, *The Rebirth of Nature: The Greening of Science and God* (New York: Bantam Books, 1992).

8. Again Toffler, *The Third Wave* (New York: Bantam Doubleday Dell, 1981), pp. 263-264. For two different perspectives (one Marxian, the other ecological) on the primacy of culture in the new stage, see Fredric Jameson, *Postmodernism, or, The Cultural Logic of Late Capitalism* (Durham: Duke University, 1992), and again Swimme & Berry, *Universe Story*, pp. 251-252.

9. See, for example, the 1995 pastoral letter of the 25 Catholic bishops of Appalachia in the United States, *At Home in the Web of Life: Sustainable Communities in Appalachia* (available from the Catholic Committee of Appalachia, PO Box 662, Webster Springs, West Virginia 26288, USA). On the more general concept of "sustainable development," see what is popularly referred to as the "Brundtland Report" by the United Nation's World Commission on Environment and Development (chaired by Gro Harlem Brundtland of Norway), *Our Common Future* (New York: Oxford University Press). See also Lester W. Milbrath, *Envisioning a Sustainable Society: Learning Our Way Out* (Albany, New York: State University of New York, 1989); Lester R. Brown, *Building a Sustainable Society* (New York: W.W. Norton, 1981); Herman E. Daly, & John B. Cobb, Jr., *For the Common Good: Redirecting the Economy toward Community, the Environment, and a Sustainable Future* (Boston: Beacon, 1989); and Brown et al., *Saving the Planet: How to Shape an Environmentally Sustainable Global Economy* (New York: W.W. Norton, 1991).

10. Perhaps the futurist who most stresses the electronic side of this projection is Alvin Toffler. See again his *The Third Wave*, especially Chapter 16, where he discusses the "electronic cottage." On the principle of bioregionalism, see Thomas Berry, *Dream of the Earth*, pp. 67-68, 163-179.

11. Again see Toffler, *Third Wave*, pp. 191, where he speaks of a new mode of production, and 192-207; also Rudolf Bahro, *Building the Green Movement* (Philadelphia: New Society, 1986); E.F. Schumacher, *Small is Beautiful: Economics as if People Mattered* (New York: Harper & Row, 1973), especially pp. 191-225; George McRobie, *Small is Possible* (New York: Harper & Row, 1981).

12. These projections are drawn from conversations with futurist Clement Bezold, President of the Institute for Alternative Futures, Arlington, Virginia, USA.

13. On the legal development of institutions of world order, see Richard A. Falk & Saul H. Mendlovitz, eds., *The Strategy of World Order*, Vols. 1-4 (New York: World Law Fund, 1966).

14. On the theory of creative chaos, see Ilya Prigogine & Isabelle Stengers, *Order out of Chaos: Man's New Dialogue with Nature* (New York: Bantam, 1984).

15. For an analysis of this shift from mass parties to networks of grass-roots movements, see the analysis of Brazilian sociologist Luis Alberto Gomez de Souza, *A actualidade da estrutura flexivel das CEB's* (Rio de Janeiro: Centro Joao XXIII, 1992).

16. I find the Hutterites of particular interest since, while North American family farms following the industrial capitalist model of agriculture (based on petrochemicals) have been rapidly failing in large numbers for some time now, the Hutterites are rapidly developing new rural colonies across the Great Plains of North America (in Canada and the United States). I became aware of this development through work with rural Catholic dioceses and religious orders in the Great Plains of Canada and the United States. For background on the Hutterites, see Peter H. Stephenson, *The Hutterian People: Ritual Rebirth in the Evolution of Communal Life* (Lanham, Maryland: University Press of America, 1991).

17. See Chapters 5 and 6 of Lester Brown et al., *Saving the Planet.*

18. See Chapter 3 of Brown et al., *Saving the Planet.*

19. See again McRobie, *Small is Possible.*

20. Such a spirituality is addressed in my book, *Creative Communion: Toward a Spirituality of Work* (New York: Paulist Press, 1989).

REFERENCES

Bahro, R. (1986). *Building the green movement.* Philadelphia: New Society.

Bellah, R. (1966). *Habits of the heart: Individualism and commitment in American life.* University of California Press.

Berry, T. (1988). The *dream of the earth.* San Francisco: Sierra Club.

Brown, L. (1981). *Building a sustainable society.* New York: W.W. Norton.

Catholic Committee of Appalachia. (1995). *At home in the web of life: Sustainable communities in Appalachia.* Webster Springs, West Virginia.

Falk, R.A., & Mendlovitz, S.H. (1966). *The strategy of world order,* Vols. 1-4. New York: World Law Fund.

Gomez de Souza, L.A. (1992). *A actualidade da estrutura flexivel das CEB's.* Rio de Janeiro: Centro Joao XXIII.

Holland, J. (1989). *Creative communion: Toward a spirituality of work.* New York: Paulist Press.

Holland, J. (1992). *The Postmodern electronic era: Myth, sexual symbol, and technological function*. Washington DC: The Warwick Institute.
Jameson, F. (1992). *Postmodernism*. Durham: Duke University.
McRobie, G. (1981). *Small is possible*. New York: Harper & Row.
Prigogine, I., & Stengers, I. (1984). *Order out of chaos: Man's new dialogue with nature*. New York: Bantam.
Schumacher, E.F. (1973). *Small is beautiful: Economics as if people mattered*. New York: Harper & Row.
Sheldrake, R. (1992). *The rebirth of nature: The greening of science and God*. New York: Bantam Books.
Spretnak, C. (1986). *The spiritual dimension of green politics*. Santa Fe, New Mexico: Bear & Co.
Stephenson, P.H. (1991). *The Hutterian people: Ritual rebirth in the evolution of communal life*. Lanham, Maryland: University Press of America.
Toffler, A. (1992). *The Third wave*. New York: William Morrow.

Developing Compassionate Communities Through the Power of Caregiving Relationships

Discussion of Professor Joe Holland's "The Regeneration of Ecological, Societal, and Spiritual Life: The Holistic Postmodern Mission of Humanity in the Newly Emerging Planetary Civilization."

Katherine Tyson

SUMMARY. To bring about compassionate communities, helping professionals need robust understandings of human nature and how humans acquire stable self-regulation and self-worth. Intrapsychic humanism's discoveries about human development, the nature of psychopathology, and an effective therapeutic process make it possible to offer effective treatments and to effectively treat people heretofore mislabeled 'untreatable.' These discoveries show how caregiving relationships (between caregivers and children and between clients and helpers) enable individuals to develop their innate motive for stable self-regulation of their motives and their well-being, so they can in turn be partners in bringing about compassionate, healing communities. *[Article copies available for a fee from The Haworth Document Delivery Service: 1-800-HAWORTH. E-mail address: <docdelivery@haworthpress.com> Website: <http://www.HaworthPress.com> © 2005 by The Haworth Press, Inc. All rights reserved.]*

Katherine Tyson, PhD, is Professor, Loyola University of Chicago School of Social Work, 820 North Michigan Avenue, Chicago, IL 60611 (E-mail: ktyson@luc.edu).

[Haworth co-indexing entry note]: "Developing Compassionate Communities Through the Power of Caregiving Relationships." Tyson, Katherine. Co-published simultaneously in *Journal of Religion & Spirituality in Social Work: Social Thought* (The Haworth Social Work Practice Press, an imprint of The Haworth Press, Inc.) Vol. 24, No. 1/2, 2005, pp. 27-33; and: *Social Work and Divinity* (ed: Daniel Lee, and Robert O'Gorman) The Haworth Social Work Practice Press, an imprint of The Haworth Press, Inc., 2005, pp. 27-33. Single or multiple copies of this article are available for a fee from The Haworth Document Delivery Service [1-800-HAWORTH, 9:00 a.m. - 5:00 p.m. (EST). E-mail address: docdelivery@haworthpress.com].

http://www.haworthpress.com/web/JRSSW

Digital Object Identifier: 10.1300/J377v24n01_03

KEYWORDS. Intrapsychic humanism, human development, caregiving, well-being, compassionate communities

This conference focuses on the importance for social workers, pastors, and theologians of developing unified responses to the social problems generated in what Professor Holland termed the modern era–social inequalities, discrimination, violence, family abuse, alienation, and loss of community. As Professor Holland says, these problems originate in oppressive aspects of modern industrialized societies. He advances a vision of a world in which communities have significantly ameliorated these problems. My response will address a question Professor Holland raises and identifies as most central of all: how scientific innovations can "enhance" rather than "diminish the planetary community of life" (p. 6).[1]

By compassionate communities I mean communities in which peace is made possible by the fulfillment of justice (Gutierrez, 1973; King, 1991; Russell, 1974). To be able to nurture compassionate communities, humans need to have a sufficient capacity for self-regulation of self-worth, stable competence in choosing and pursuing goals, and caring treatment of others. The scientific discoveries that shed light on how humans can develop stable self-regulation are the technologies available for bringing about communities based on a just social order–these discoveries are the focus here.

Contemporary developmental psychology indicates that many prior theories about human nature and caregiving relationships are no longer the best ways to understand human development, the origins of human psychological disorder, and the process of healing or treatment. As leading child development researchers such as Andrew Meltzoff (Gopnik & Meltzoff, 1997), Colwyn Trevarthan (Trevarthan & Aitken, 2001), and Martha and William Pieper point out (Pieper & Pieper, 1990), it is generally agreed that current discoveries undercut social learning theory and central principles of both Piaget's theory of cognitive development, and also Freudian psychoanalytic theory and its derivatives in the works of Mahler and Winnicott.

Instead, contemporary child development researchers and brain scientists (e.g., Sperry, 1982, 1993) increasingly confirm the view of human nature set forth in the innovative psychology and philosophy of mind, intrapsychic humanism. This viewpoint recognizes that humans are motivated most powerfully to actualize their ideals of self-regulation and to experience compassionate relationship pleasure, and specifically that the caregiving relationships that exist between parents and children and between clients and therapists are the most powerful influences that shape humans' self-regulatory capacity. This view of human nature was discovered in the 1970s by Martha Heineman Pieper, a clinical social worker, and William Joseph Pieper, a child and adult psychoanalyst (Pieper & Pieper, 1990, 1995, 1999). Intrapsychic humanism is a comprehensive theory of child development, psychopathology, and treatment, grounded in humanistic values, and free of biases based on gender, race, sexual orientation, socioeconomic status, and status of disability. It offers guidelines for effective treatment of all people with all psychological disorders, from all cultures, using all modalities (e.g., individual, family, group, residential), and a compassionate approach to parenting that both helps parents enjoy parenting and also raise more competent, happy, and caring children (Pieper & Pieper, 1999).

Findings from the international community of child development researchers in experimental laboratories (e.g., Colwyn Trevarthan in Edinburgh and Andrew Meltzoff in the United States) are supporting the discoveries of intrapsychic humanism. Consider for examples the following: (1) From the moment a human becomes conscious, s/he experiences an overridingly powerful motive to regulate her/himself based on her/his relationship experience with caregivers. A fetus in the womb will turn towards the sound of it's mother's voice; newborns can distinguish their parents from all other adults, even at birth and they will move their arms and legs to the rhythm of their parents' voices; (2) Children's self-regulation occurs by internalizing their relationship experience with caregivers and treating themselves as they have been treated; they internalize and imitate not just behavior, but even more importantly, intentionality (Pieper & Pieper, 1990). Experimental laboratories have found that children as young as five months old reliably discriminate purposeful and non-purposeful behavior (Woodward, 1999), and 18-month-old infants can distinguish between the behavior and the intentionality of their caregivers (Meltzoff, 1995); (3) Children as young as 18-months-old have been observed to try to soothe their emotionally distressed parents (Kempe and Helfer, 1980), and three year-old children have a sophisticated understanding of relationships and emotions and will try to conform their own emotions to suit the needs of their caregivers (Banerjee, 1997). In other words, children develop their experience of their own motives (their identity) based on their experience of what their parents want for them and need from them (Pieper & Pieper, 1990). Finally, (4) many of the behaviors and emotions thought to be unavoidable, normal aspects of child development–such as the 'terrible twos,' temper tantrums, and nightmares–are preventable through specific child-rearing practices, whereas other child behaviors thought to indicate a 'difficult' temperament or an 'at-risk' child can be transitory if responded to facilitatively by parents and other caregivers (Pieper & Pieper, 1990, 1999).

Intrapsychic humanism had its first formal public expression in a pioneering project that provided inpatient and residential care to teenage state wards of the Illinois Department of Children and Family Services whose homicidally and suicidally violent behavior made it impossible to house them anywhere other than a locked inpatient unit, and had led other care providers to deem them incurable (1995). These teenagers had been labeled mentally retarded as well as psychotic. Their future, like that of many others suffering the combination of abuse, neglect, and stigma, would have been tragic–early violent deaths or the back wards of institutions for the criminally insane. Within a relatively brief period of time–2 1/2 years–the systematic application of the principles of intrapsychic humanism made it possible to safely house the teenagers in an unlocked residential group home, and demonstrated that they in fact were not mentally retarded by integrating them into mainstream classrooms. Most importantly, this project demonstrated that even those deemed most out of reach of psychological healing, and those most prone to commit crimes commonly regarded as heinous, still possess the motivation to benefit from an intrapsychic caregiving relationship to develop their capacity for healthy self-regulation.

The remarkable changes in these adolescents were made possible by the most important discovery of intrapsychic humanism–intrapsychic consciousness. Innate but then requiring confirmation from a caregiving relationship, the motive generated by intrapsychic consciousness makes it possible for humans to acquire genuine self-regulation when their caregivers give the cared-for individual the experience that s/he can cause her/his caregivers to love and care for her/him. Beginning at birth, every human is most powerfully motivated to develop an autonomous mind organized by the caregiving relationship available with her/his parents. Optimally, by the end of the third year of life, the caregiving relationship has given children a stable mental structure of intrapsychic self-regulation. This structure makes it possible for children to have an autonomous wellspring of inner well-being that is also the basis for accurate self-knowledge, competent self-caretaking, and compassionate treatment of others (Pieper & Pieper, 1990, 1999).

Intrapsychic humanism's understanding of human nature recognizes that humans truly cannot live by bread alone (Pieper & Pieper, 1990).

Humans are not born with endogenous motives for hatred or destructiveness, but in fact are born loving their caregivers, as is expressed in the smile that lights up the face of human infants at the sight of their caregiver's face. If the infant's innate motive is responded to by veridical caregiving love, the "I" of the emergent self that the caregiving mutuality brings into existence consists of a "we-ness" that affords an enduring capacity to bring about a meaningful experience of personal existence–the individual's capacity for self-regulatory control of the self, which includes competence and a genuine capacity for love.

Intrapsychic consciousness is so powerful that it can actually regulate aspects of human physiological functioning, which explains syndromes such as failure to thrive or marasmus, anorexia, and suicide, in which the individual sacrifices her/his physiological well-being and even survival to preserve a sense of intrapsychic well-being (Pieper & Pieper, 1990). When the infant or child is deprived of the reflection from a caregiver that is adequate for intrapsychic development, s/he will withdraw internally to a starter supply of intrapsychic personal meaning, sacrificing contact with the external world, and even food and physical survival. Children who receive sufficient relationship experience to survive, but who are subjected to violence or emotional abuse, will unknowingly attach the meaning of ideal care to those abusive experiences, seeking actively to recreate the abuse in caring for her/himself and others, and in effect acquiring self-destructive motives for self-caused unhappiness. In other words, "Children become mentally ill out of love for their parents" (Pieper & Pieper, 1999).

Fortunately, intrapsychic humanism treatment can ameliorate many physiological syndromes that have been caused or exacerbated by suboptimal nurture, ranging from psychosocial dwarfism to childhood asthma. Many conditions commonly thought to be based in some organic defect in the child, such as childhood hyperactivity and many learning disabilities, can be cured through psychotherapy based on the principles of intrapsychic humanism (Tyson, 1991, 1994, 1998, 2000). Healing is possible because clients bring to their therapists the same innate motive to acquire self-regulation through causing the caregiver's caregiving. Because the therapist's nurture will offer better intrapsychic gratification than the abusive intimacy to which the client had to become attached, this original intrapsychic motive can be elicited and strengthened by treatment based on the principles of intrapsychic humanism. Moreover, for the many people who are not raised in the embrace of genuine caregiving love or whose families, despite their efforts to care for the children, are devastated by war or disaster, the nature of the communities in which they then reside makes all the difference for their development. The more compassion individuals experience in their communities, the more individuals can be supported in foregoing self-destructive motives and developing the motives for constructive self-regulation with which they were born (Tyson & Carroll, 2001).

In conclusion, of all the technological advances we have seen, the advances in our understanding of developmental caregiving relationships–specifically the relationship that exists between parents and children, and the caregiving relationship created between those engaged in therapeutic activities an those seeking psychological healing–are critically important for the meaning of our own lives and for the development of compassionate communities. The healing power of care- giving relationships can bring about the satisfaction of our quest for a life that is meaningful and that fulfills our most cherished ideals of developing a just social order. Just as importantly, these new discoveries include guidelines for offering our children and those who come to us for psychological help, caregiving relationships that provide the self-regulation that is their birthright, and that enables them to be partners in establishing a compassionate communities.

NOTE

References to Professor Holland's paper cite the pagination of the draft reviewed in April, 2002.

REFERENCES

Banerjee, M. (1997). Hidden emotions: Preschoolers' knowledge of appearance-reality and emotion display rules. *Social Cognition 15*, 107-132.

Gopnik, A., and A. Meltzoff (1997). *Words, thoughts, and theories*. Cambridge, MA: MIT Press.

Gutierrez, G. (1973). *A theology of liberation: History, politics, and salvation*. Maryknoll, NY: Orbis Books.

Kempe, C. H., and R. E. Helfer (1980). *The battered child, 3rd edition revised and expanded*. Chicago: University of Chicago Press.

King, M. L., Jr. (1991). *A testament of hope: The essential writings and speeches of Martin Luther King, Jr*. San Francisco: 1st Harper Collins.

Meltzoff, A. (1995). Understanding the intentions of others: Re-enactment of intended acts by 18-month-old children. *Developmental Psychology 31*, 838-850.

Pieper, M. H., and W. J. Pieper (1990). *Intrapsychic humanism: An introduction to a comprehensive psychology and philosophy of mind*. Chicago: Falcon II Press. For further information about intrapsychic humanism, see also *www.intrapsychichumanism.com*

Pieper, M. H., and W. J. Pieper (1995). Treating violent, 'untreatable' adolescents: Applications of intrapsychic humanism in a state-funded demonstration project. In K. Tyson (Ed.), *New foundations for scientific social and behavioral research: The heuristic paradigm*. Needham Heights, MA: Allyn & Bacon.

Pieper, M. H., and W.J. Pieper. (1999). *Smart love: The compassionate alternative to discipline that will make you a better parent and your child a better person*. Boston: Harvard Common Press.

Russell, L. M. (1974). *Human liberation in a feminist perspective: A theology*. Philadelphia: Westminster Press.

Simpson, J. A., and E. S. C. Weinder (1991). *The Compact Oxford English Dictionary, Second Edition*. Oxford: Clarendon Press.

Sperry, R. (1982). Some effects of disconnecting the cerebral hemispheres. *Science 217*, 1223-1225.

Sperry, R. W. (1993). The impact and promise of the cognitive revolution. *American Psychologist 48*, 878-885.

Trevarthan, C., and K. J. Aitken (2001). Infant intersubjectivity: Research, theory, and clinical applications. *Journal of Child Psychology and Psychiatry 42*(1): 3-48.

Tyson, K. (1991). The understanding and treatment of childhood hyperactivity: Old problems and new approaches. *Smith College Studies in Social Work 61*, 133-166.

Tyson, K. (1994). Heuristic guidelines for naturalistic qualitative evaluations of child treatment. In E. Sherman and W.J. Reid (Eds.), *Qualitative research in social work*. New York: Columbia University Press.

Tyson, K. (1998). Therapy from the child's perspective. Invitational Honorary Alumni Address, Loyola University of Chicago, Chicago, IL.

Tyson, K. (2000). Using the teacher-student relationship to help children diagnosed as hyperactive. *Child and Youth Care Forum 29*, 265-289.

Tyson, K., and E. Carroll (2001). Innovative therapeutic care for homeless, severely mentally ill clients: Intrapsychic humanism in a residential setting. *Families in Society: Journal of the Contemporary Human Services 82*, 591-603.

Woodward, A. (1999). Infants' ability to distinguish between purposeful and non-purposeful behaviors. *Infant Behavior and Development 22*, 145-160.

Issues, Components, and Theoretical Considerations in the Integration of Divinity and Social Work Curricula

Homer U. Ashby, Jr.

SUMMARY. This article describes the common and distinctive features of Divinity and Social Work Curricula. The investigation of these curricula includes an examination of the theoretical foundations of each discipline, program design, field work options, and the need for joint planning. The suggestion is made that dual degree be dropped as the nomenclature for such cooperative programs and that they be named joint degrees programs. *[Article copies available for a fee from The Haworth Document Delivery Service: 1-800-HAWORTH. E-mail address: <docdelivery@haworthpress.com> Website: <http://www.HaworthPress.com> © 2005 by The Haworth Press, Inc. All rights reserved.]*

Homer U. Ashby, Jr., PhD, is W. Clement and Jessie V. Stone Professor of Pastoral Care at McCormick Theological Seminary. He holds a BA from Princeton University, a MTh and a DMin from the University of Chicago, and a PhD from Garrett Evangelical Theological Seminary/Northwestern University.

Address correspondence to: Homer U. Ashby, Jr., PhD, McCormick Theological Seminary, 5555 South Woodlawn Avenue, Chicago, IL 60637 (E-mail: hashby@mccormick. edu).

[Haworth co-indexing entry note]: "Issues, Components, and Theoretical Considerations in the Integration of Divinity and Social Work Curricula."Ashby, Homer U., Jr. Co-published simultaneously in *Journal of Religion & Spirituality in Social Work: Social Thought* (The Haworth Social Work Practice Press, an imprint of The Haworth Press, Inc.) Vol. 24, No. 1/2, 2005, pp. 35-44; and: *Social Work and Divinity* (ed: Daniel Lee, and Robert O'Gorman) The Haworth Social Work Practice Press, an imprint of The Haworth Press, Inc., 2005, pp. 35-44. Single or multiple copies of this article are available for a fee from The Haworth Document Delivery Service [1-800-HAWORTH, 9:00 a.m. - 5:00 p.m. (EST). E-mail address: docdelivery@haworthpress.com].

http://www.haworthpress.com/web/JRSSW

Digital Object Identifier: 10.1300/J377v24n01_04

KEYWORDS. Divinity school curriculum, social work curriculum, dual degree programs, cooperative professional programs, end of life issues

INTRODUCTION

The integration of divinity and social work curricula has both a practical side and a theoretical side. The practical side has to do with number of credit hours, sequencing of courses, coordinating field work, etc. The theoretical side has to do with the relationship between theology and social work theory, dual professional identity, the aims and expected outcomes of the practice of ministry and the practice of social work. The best programs that integrate the two sets of curricula take both sides seriously. And in considering both sides do so in a mutually influencing way as opposed to the railroad track model. In the railroad track model the two separate tracks run side by side connected by buried ties, but never crossing. In fact their crossing or inability to maintain a certain distance from one another can lead to tragedy. In the not too distant past this was the fear held by both divinity and social work. For social work the introduction of religion and/or spirituality tainted the possibility to do effective and authentic social work. For divinity too much emphasis on social work failed to address the soul and could lead to a kind of works righteousness. For the most part those days have passed and we have entered into a time in which there is an interest, even appreciation, for the role each of these disciplines can play in enhancing the quality of life for persons. Yet, there is still a need for greater clarity about how to best construct a mutually influencing model of religion and social work.

This article begins with an identification of all of the practical issues and concerns that are associated with dual degree programs. Next, I want to reflect on some of the theoretical issues that arise in the midst of the conflation of these two disciplines. And finally I will return to the practical issues in light of the theoretical concerns so as to suggest a model for how to integrate the curricula of divinity and social work. First the practical issues.

DUAL PROGRAM DESIGN

Any professional degree program is trying to do three things: (1) introduce students to the profession; its history, its values, its assumptions, its distinctiveness as a field; (2) teach students the theory and skills necessary for effective work in the profession; and (3) engage students in formation activities that contribute to the creation of a professional identity in that profession. Each of the two disciplines we are discussing here do this by offering courses and other learning activities, arranging field work opportunities and providing events, space and encouragement to participate in disciplines that shape the student as a person and as a professional. The courses are usually arranged in a particular sequence, whereby knowledge builds upon knowledge. Beginning with foundational courses, students take more advanced and elective courses that rest on that solid foundation. It is generally expected that students will have acquired a certain basic level of knowledge and perhaps skill set so as to be ready to enter into the practice of their profession. Field work is done under supervision. The supervision does two things minimally. The supervisor guides the student in how to be a practitioner in the profession and is a model of how to carry out the responsibilities and tasks associated with the profession. Praxis or reflection on practice occurs throughout the course of study. Whether through case studies in theory classes, or critical reflection on an actual intervention, students are trained to be reflective observers of the exercise of their ministry or social work. These elements in the preparation of men and women for the two professions are common to both.

Where there begins to be some diversity or difference is how the two programs work together to create this mutually enhancing curriculum. Which school does a student start with first: divinity or social work? Does it make a difference? Will starting in one school skew the student's professional loyalties to one profession more so than the other? Is there something intrinsic about theological study or social work that make it important that a student begin with one, to be followed by the other?

Most theological schools are three-year programs. Most social work schools are two-year programs. What should be the sequential structure of these two programs? Should it be 2a-2b-1a? Or 1a-2b-1a? Or 2a-3b? Or 3a-2b? Or 1a-1b-2a-1b? Or 1a-1b-1a-2b? Or 1a-1b-1a-1b-1a? Does it make a difference? Does either of these sequences improve integration between the programs?

And what about field work? Can there be a field work site that satisfies both schools' requirements for field work? Does field work in one discipline necessarily create conflict in the student in another discipline because of conflicting professional development expectations? Is supervision from a theological perspective different from supervision from a social work perspective? These questions associated with the practical elements of dual degree programs point to real and important questions and issues on the theoretical side.

DUAL DEGREE PROGRAM THEORETICAL PERSPECTIVES

There are many theoretical issues that can be explored when looking at the theoretical side of the dual degree discourse. For purpose of this article the one theoretical issue that I would like to investigate is that of the aims of the professions; that is the aim of social work and the aim of ministry. Again as in the case of the practical side I believe that there are common elements in the theoretical dimensions of social work and ministry as well as differentiating features. I think it is safe to say that each of these professions professes that it is committed to the health and well being of individuals and communities. Each of these professions seeks to bring its own particular body of knowledge, skills and values to bear on the human condition so as to change or transform persons and systems so that they better conform to the profession's vision of health and wholeness. I think a third common element is a need to be informed by other disciplines so as to effect change, transformation, health and wholeness in the most effective and comprehensive manner. There may indeed be other common elements, but these are the primary ones that I want to introduce now.

When it comes to differentiating features I think there is one that is primary: an orientation toward a life of faith. Social work and ministry both recognize the life of faith as a dimension of healthy and whole living, but social work and ministry think differently about their roles in fostering the life of faith. When it comes to the life of faith social work tends to be more descriptive and ministry tends to be more prescriptive. Social work tends to recognize the presence of a transcendent other, while ministry tends to push for a kind of relationship with the transcendent other. In social work spirituality tends more to be a practice or discipline, whereas in ministry spirituality is more a way of life. Finally, in social work the life of faith is viewed as resource while in ministry the life of faith is an affirmation of faith that one lives into. In order to clarify the distinctions that I have made above I would like to examine a particular life event from the theoretical perspective of social work and ministry. That life event is end of life.

In a very helpful and useful book published by the American Cancer Society, four social workers discuss social work in oncology (Lauria et al., 2001). In a chapter entitled, "End of Life Issues," they discuss spirituality at the end of life:

> Spirituality goes beyond readily defined social roles and relationships (Sharp, 1997) and focuses on one's relationship with the inner "self" or the "soul" as well as with the possibility of a life or existence beyond the finite world. Relationships with others, God, and the universes may be of concern as death approaches and the question of meaning becomes paramount. (p. 307)

They go on to further state regarding grief:

> Many people with life-threatening illnesses and their loved ones begin the process of grieving as their illness changes life, and with the reality that life is ending, face saying goodbye to those they love, and contend with finding meaning in life and in dying. (p. 308)

Social work recognizes that a relationship with that which transcends sense phenomena is a *possibility* and *may* be a part of the person's grieving process. The tentative language that social work employs when making reference to things spiritual makes sense. Social workers are not trained nor are they expected to make pronouncements about faith. In ministry, pastors are expected to make a strong declaration about how faith matters are at the heart of end of life issues. Kenneth Mitchell and Herbert Anderson, pastoral theologians, have this to say about grieving: "In the church, care for mourners is undergirded by the confidence that the future is secure in the promise of God" (Mitchell and Anderson, 1983, p. 108). Their theology of grieving claims that:

> Our understanding of the pervasiveness of loss is organized around the conviction that finitude is part of the creation which God regarded as good. Finitude, including the physical death of our flesh, is a necessary part of the orderliness of life. (p. 163)

At the end of life social workers recognize and acknowledge the possible inclusion of spirituality as a resource for those who grieve. Making meaning at the end of life may benefit from a relationship with the transcendent other and the disciplines associated with the maintenance of that relationship. For ministers spirituality is a necessary part of end of life process. In ministry the pastor seeks to help the dying person and their loved ones make faith affirmations about life and death and live those affirmations. Some of the interventions associated with their role as religious leader include prayer, worship or ritual coordinator, pastoral counselor, and spiritual director.

What are the roles and interventions of social workers at the end of life? Lauria and her colleagues state that the social worker assumes the following roles with patients and families: "evaluator, counselor, educator, advocate, case manager, group worker, discharge planner, and liaison to hospital and community resources" (Lauria et al., 2001, p. 146). In fulfilling these roles the social worker will engage in the following interventions:

- Incorporating psychosocial services into coordinated, comprehensive care programs;
- Offering continuity of psychosocial care to all patients and families from diagnosis through treatment and into extended survivorship or bereavement;
- Sharing responsibility for psychosocial care among multidisciplinary team members;
- Offering a wide range of clinical services, such as advocacy, supportive counseling, and other therapies, behavioral interventions, stress management, education, and resource provision and referral;
- Providing varied support programs, such as parent, sibling, or other support groups, school re-entry programs, summer camps, buddy programs, recreational activities, bereavement groups, and survivor programs;
- Using medical center volunteers in special programs to supplement the work of psychosocial professionals;
- Collaborating with community and national voluntary health and other organizations to expand psychosocial care through shared programs and initiatives (Lauria et al., 2001, pages 145-146).

In essence, social workers focus on psychosocial care while ministers focus on pastoral care. It can be seen that there may be some overlap in role and function, but the distinguishing differentiation is between the focus of the two kinds of care: psychosocial support and growth in faith. This does not mean that social workers may not be interested in issues of faith or that ministers are not interested in psychosocial issues. Rather the two professions have a joint interest in health and wholeness of persons and in their efforts to secure that health and wholeness focus their knowledge, skills and practice in some similar, but also distinct ways.

DUAL DEGREE CURRICULA

What does all of this have to do with dual degree curricula in divinity and social work? When I first contemplated this question I thought I would work with the notion that there are four models of divinity social work integration:

1. Ministry with social work knowledge and skills;
2. A Ministry of social work;
3. Social work with a religious or spiritual component;
4. Social Work as ministry.

I was then going to define each of these models, demarcating their similarities and differences. The thrust of my thinking about theses models was to challenge divinity and social work schools that are in dual degree programs with one another to choose which model they operated out of and to assist students in their appropriation of that model. Along the way I was going to describe how to design a curriculum that reflected the different models. As I entered into the process of writing this article I decided to jettison that approach. Let me explain why.

The fact that these different models may exist is, in part, the result of a lack of clarity about the nature and intent of dual degree programs in divinity and social work. Many of the students who come through our program are not always clear about the integration of these two degree programs. Different students come out with different understandings of the integration both personally and professionally. Now perhaps that should be seen as a good thing in that there may indeed be a variety of ways of thinking about and formulating dual degree programs with these two disciplines so that students have a choice in what model they will employ in their life and work. However, I came to the conclusion that the variety of models was the result not of a dynamic synergism between these two disciplines, but the inability of professional schools in divinity and social work to be clear with one another about what they are doing with dual degree programs.

I was aided in my change of thought by the experience of a couple of current students who brought to our school's attention the absence of a clear curricular theory of integration that undergirded their courses of study. Each student is enrolled in a different school of social work that has adopted two different approaches to coursework. One school requires that each dual degree student complete all of the courses in its social work curriculum. In the other school dual degree students can apply some of their divinity course work to meet course requirements in the social work school. On what basis does the one school accept transfer credit and the other school not? This is not clear in our school and neither is it clear to us why we support both kinds of arrangements. Are we saying that there are different ways of integrating the two curricula or are we just supporting two different curricula options without critical examination? I am afraid to admit that it is more the latter than the former.

So where does that leave us? And how do we approach the problem? I think the first thing that we ought to do is drop the language of "dual degree program." Referring back to my earlier analogy of two train tracks, dual degree suggests that the two curricula run side by side, but are only indirectly associated with one another. We should be creating "joint degrees programs." Joint degrees helps move in the direction of better integration in the curriculum. First of all a joint degrees program would mean that both schools would sit down and hammer out what are the basic assumptions, values, course requirements and curricular implications of training persons in both divinity and social work. It would not be left up to the student by him or herself to discern the interdisciplinary rationale that underlies the curriculum. Nor would the two schools run the risk of working from two different understandings about what it means to form persons with knowledge, skills and values in the two disciplines. The common understandings about basic assumptions about the joint program would lead to the design of a curriculum that both schools owned. Moreover, the common understandings about how the two disciplines are joined in a mutually adopted model would lead to curriculum design that reflected those common understandings. Indeed there may be different models of integration that are out there, but with joint planning and design the multitude of options would not be found in the confusing array of integration options with which students graduate, but would be found in the array of models two schools would choose as the integration model that reflects their joint thinking, planning, and curriculum design.

Thus all questions about curriculum design would flow from this joint planning. Some examples: Traditionally, social work school programs for a full-time student are two years long. For theological seminaries they are usually three years long for a full-time student. At our school now a student does two years in divinity and we transfer a year of social work school to make up the third year of the divinity degree. Is this the best way to integrate when it comes to curricular design? And in this arrangement we offer flexibility to the student in how they might want to locate themselves at the two schools. At our school right now the standard arrangements are two years at our school and two years at social work school. Another option that exists is one year at our school, two years in social work school, and one year back at our school. Two other options exist, but are less frequently employed: (1) two years at social work school and two years at our school, and (2) one year at social work school, two years at our school and one year at social work school. Students choose which option they desire. Might not there be a preferred arrangement based upon what kind of personal and professional identity we want students to achieve? Critical thinking about the kind of integration we want to see take place might better determine the preferred arrangement other than just student choice. Given what has been presented above I would certainly suggest that a student spend a concentrated period of time at both schools, rather than go back and forth. In this way the student has a chance to more successfully be formed in both disciplines. Whether one begins with social work or divinity I think makes little difference.

What about field work? Our school requires one year of field work. Most social work schools require two years. One school with whom we have a dual degree program will allow certain of our field work placements to satisfy one of their placements. Another partner school does not. On what basis does the one school allow this and the other not? Does it serve integration of curriculum better or worse to have joint field work placements? This is a question that needs to be thought through with intentionality in order to design curriculum that serves both professions and schools well. More important than the field work site arrangements is the supervisor. In a joint degrees program field work placement the supervisor should be a person who has a joint professional identity; that is, a person who has either graduated from a joint degrees program or has graduated from both degree programs, but not in a joint program. In such a field site with such a supervisor the student has a ready model of how to function out of the shared professional identities.

At our school we offer an integration seminar throughout the year to assist in the integration process. At times the seminar has been required for graduation, at other times not. At times the seminar has been given academic credit, at other times not. The number of times the seminar has been held throughout the year has varied; sometimes once a month, other times once a quarter. Any one of these arrangements might be just fine, but the integrity of the arrangement is based upon a thoughtful consideration of what is sought in integration and how integration takes place. Again discussions between the two schools on these topics will result in a curricular model that will reflect the basic assumptions and joint thinking of the two schools. My own recommendation is that there be a required credit bearing course to which each school gives credit, taught by resident faculty of the two schools, whose principle aim is to assist students in the integration of divinity and social work.

CONCLUSION

Theoretically, joint degree programs should clarify the assumptions shared by the two disciplines as well as distinguish the assumptions that differentiate them. Where there is conflict students should be helped to recognize the areas of tension and given tools with which to practically and theoretically manage the conflict. In order to demonstrate common and collective ownership by both schools the leadership of the joint degree seminar should rotate among faculty members of both schools.

The existence of dual degree programs in divinity and social work have the potential to produce dedicated professionals whose expertise in two fields can dramatically increase the contribution they can make to the health and wholeness of persons and the well-being of society. If schools that offer these programs can see themselves working more jointly rather than separately they will not only enhance the quality of the educational experience, but also lend integrity to their programs.

REFERENCES

Lauria, M. M., Clark, E. J., Hermann, J. F., & Stearns, N. M. (2001). *Social work in oncology: Supporting survivors, families, and caregivers.* Atlanta, GA: American Cancer Society.

Mitchell, K. R., & Anderson, H. (1983). *All our losses, all our grieves: Resources for pastoral care.* Philadelphia: Westminster Press.

The Role of Religion and Spirituality in Clinical Social Work: Creating a Space for Integration in MSW/MDiv Joint Programs

Terry B. Northcut

SUMMARY. Social work has a history of treating the whole person in his/her environment, however, the effort to be scientific in our approach to clinical practice often has obscured our examination of the religious and spiritual beliefs and practices of our clients and in our own lives. Consequently, there has been very little guidance to date on how curriculum can help integrate the professional identities of MSW/MDiv students. An elective practice course, "The Role of Religion and Spirituality in Clinical Social Work" in our accredited graduate social work program provides a transitional space for this integration to occur through a guiding framework of psychodynamic, systems, and postmodern theories. *[Article copies available for a fee from The Haworth Document Delivery Service: 1-800-HAWORTH. E-mail address: <docdelivery@haworthpress.com> Website: <http://www.HaworthPress.com> © 2005 by The Haworth Press, Inc. All rights reserved.]*

Terry B. Northcut, PhD, LCSW, is Associate Professor, Loyola University of Chicago, School of Social Work, 820 North Michigan Avenue, Chicago, IL 60611 (E-mail: tnorthc@wpo.it.luc.edu).

[Haworth co-indexing entry note]: "The Role of Religion and Spirituality in Clinical Social Work: Creating a Space for Integration in MSW/MDiv Joint Programs." Northcut, Terry B. Co-published simultaneously in *Journal of Religion & Spirituality in Social Work: Social Thought* (The Haworth Social Work Practice Press, an imprint of The Haworth Press, Inc.) Vol. 24, No. 1/2, 2005, pp. 45-54; and: *Social Work and Divinity* (ed: Daniel Lee, and Robert O'Gorman) The Haworth Social Work Practice Press, an imprint of The Haworth Press, Inc., 2005, pp. 45-54. Single or multiple copies of this article are available for a fee from The Haworth Document Delivery Service [1-800-HAWORTH, 9:00 a.m. - 5:00 p.m. (EST). E-mail address: docdelivery@haworthpress.com].

http://www.haworthpress.com/web/JRSSW

Digital Object Identifier: 10.1300/J377v24n01_05

KEYWORDS. Religion, spirituality, curriculum, MSW/MDIV joint degrees

INTRODUCTION

Dual degree MSW/MDiv students often are frustrated by the lack of curriculum or classroom assistance within the school of social work for integration of the two degrees. While each of the separate graduate programs have courses geared to facilitate the development of a professional identity from that discipline's vantage point, neither seems to provide space for the student attempting to balance or integrate dual identities. From a social work standpoint, we have made some changes in our curriculum that we hope will benefit the dual degree student. To begin with, the Council on Social Work Education now requires content on religion and spiritual diversity in the curriculum of accredited social work programs. What is not clearly specified is how that content should be integrated and to what extent. This paper will consider how our program attempts to integrate the two areas in our methods (clinical practice) sequence and the theoretical frameworks that support our approach.

Our social work program includes readings on religious and spiritual diversity in both human behavior and methods courses. These readings facilitate students in understanding the function of religion and spirituality in clients' lives and communities, how religion and spirituality can foster or hinder resiliency and the ways in which religion and spirituality may shape health care. In addition, our most significant effort has been the development and inclusion of a course on "the role of religion and spirituality in clinical social work." Courses on differing world religions, justice and ethics, the dynamics of faith, adult faith development and spiritual assessment, and Christian pastoral counseling are already available in the Loyola curriculum in the departments of theology and pastoral care. What we lacked in our social work program was a forum to examine in greater depth the ways in which religion and spirituality are present in the therapeutic space, and how the clinician can effectively and ethically intervene. The challenge was to how to organize the cacophony of possible frameworks.

THEORETICAL FRAMEWORK OF COURSE

Traditionally, our methods courses draw on a theoretical foundation that includes emphases on psychodynamic theory, systems theories, and our National Association of Social Work's (NASW) code of ethics to provide standards for care. These frameworks emphasize numerous variables including the following: the primacy of early development and history, the importance of self awareness, an appreciation of diversity, the principle of reciprocity (a change in one component of a system affects the other components), the importance of current research and knowledge of psychological, sociological, and biological processes, the need for critical thinking skills to evaluated this knowledge base, and the need to keep current with changes in our guiding paradigms. Sometimes these factors can create discordant notes in terms of competition for center stage in building curriculum. However, in the case of developing a course on the role of religion and spirituality in clinical social work practice, these frameworks dovetailed nicely. For example, an emphasis on the importance of understanding personal history translates easily into understanding our professional history and its' relationship to the topics of religion and spirituality. The importance of self-awareness guides us to take into consideration ethical dilemmas and countertransference issues as they contribute to what actions we do or do not take with clients. Appreciating diversity necessitates our understanding different belief systems and behavioral practices. This diversity may vary from culture to culture, family to family, and individual to individual. Consequently, an intervention on the part of a clinician to one member of a system (e.g., questioning a belief) may lead to reverberations within the family. The influence of current research shapes influences many areas of practice, including what is considered "normal" and "abnormal." Joint degree students with a MSW/ MDiv are in a position of assessing and evaluating clients in their fieldwork and must be able to assess the ways in which religious and spiritual beliefs and practices impact these clients. Drawing on quantitative and qualitative research allows practitioners to take into account the context for what is known about behavior at this point in time, and reserve room for the inevitable need to revise our ideas about what is "true" and "accurate." Postmodernism is the inevitable result of recognizing this subjectivity of our knowledge base.

Course Outline

The frameworks of psychodynamic theory, systems theory, professional ethical guidelines, and current research including postmodernism shapes the organization of our course. We set a tone from the beginning of the semester that fosters the clinician's personal awareness and development with a clear understanding of his or her own motives in examining religion and spirituality in the lives of clients. The course begins with an examination of the history of the relationship between religion and social work and the ways in which public policy is shaped by and influenced by religion. By beginning the course in this fashion, there is room for discussion of the role of social workers in advocacy and effecting social change. We then focus on professional guidelines and the values of the profession of social work. There are some inherent tensions and dilemmas manifest in trying to integrate religion/spirituality and social work. We naturally progress to developing guidelines for using spiritually based activities and working to gain comfort with the inevitable lack of clear answers in the therapeutic arena. For example, a common struggle for students is how to reconcile and work with beliefs of clients that appear to be detrimental or not best for all members of the client system; as Paul Pruyser (1977) described the often overlooked negative side of religious beliefs, "the seamy side of religious beliefs." This struggle is most evident when student clinicians confront clients with more conservative beliefs than their own. However, this conflict can also manifest as the countertransference reaction described as "my way is Yahweh" (Case, 1997) by clinicians wanting clients to agree with their belief in the superiority of their own beliefs and practices.

Self-Awareness

While dual degree students usually enter the social work program with an understanding of, or at least a greater comfort with, reflecting on their own spirituality, we do require a self-awareness component in our course. This portion of the course requires students to examine the context of their own beliefs and the foundation for their commitment to personal or professional agendas for clients functioning. Such a focus provides an important segue to understanding countertransference issues with similar or different beliefs with clients. A particularly important function of this component for the dual degree student is to look at the problems inherent in dual relationships of a "therapist and a spiritual guide." Also included in this section is the clash that can occur between practitioner beliefs, theoretical orientations, and professional beliefs–particularly if there are two professional ethoses at play. For example, in social work, the value of client self-determination is a large part of the professional code of ethics. This belief may contrast with an emphasis in divinity programs about the need to acknowledge and nourish a spiritual life.

Knowledge and Appreciation of Diverse Beliefs

Understanding diverse cultural beliefs, values, and practices is key for clinical social workers. Dual degree students may have had exposure to a variety of world religions, however in this social work course the focus is on diverse practice interventions with these varied religious/spiritual beliefs. Student cases are utilized to demonstrate and problem solve around how to choose the means to effectively intervene in ways that are consistent with the social work code of ethics and sound practice principles. For example, a recent student struggled around the issue of helping a child understand the death of a parent. The student's dilemma was assessing the degree to which the beliefs expressed by the child were helpful to the child and consistent with the family's belief system as opposed to a belief that was causing internal distress. The inevitable dilemma was whether and how to respond in a manner different from the parents. If the child were assisted in believing in an afterlife, for example, that was counter to parental beliefs, emotional distress for the child and the family would result. The student had to be assisted in remaining mindful of the impact on the larger system as well as the immediate impact of her responses to the child.

Models of Faith and Spirituality

Developmental models of faith and/or spirituality are more familiar to divinity students. And while these are studied as well, we try to move away from a linear approach to understanding spirituality and focus instead on a variety of ways of understanding spiritual issues, i.e., findings themes of ambivalence, the search for security in moral absolutes, etc. Several texts have been written regarding spiritual themes in treatment such as Fleischman's (1989) "The Healing Zone" and Cornett's (1998) "The Soul of Psychotherapy." In addition to material from these texts we use readings designed to increase students' comfort level with "feet planted firmly in midair" (Anderson, 1999), i.e., living with the paradoxes inherent in spirituality or as Cornett describes this phenomenon "comfort with chaos." One of our texts is Walsh's "Spiritual Resources in Family Therapy" (Walsh, 2001). Weingarten, an author in that edited volume, writes about "Stretching to meet what's given: Opportunities for a spiritual practice." In her discussion of the personal ways in which spirituality has shaped her practice she discusses poet John Keat's concept of "negative capability." Keats idea is that negative capability is when we are "capable of being in uncertainties, mysteries, doubts, without any irritable reaching after fact and reason." (Bate, 1963, p. 249; in Weingarten, p. 246). This is something we try to do as clinicians . . . live with this negative capability without irritable reaching. Recognizing the value of clients' rights for self-determination must extend to students in terms of avoiding trying to solve the struggles inherent in reconciling different professional roles and paradoxes in beliefs. Our psychodynamic training emphasizes the power of the relationship to facilitate growth. Likewise, the curriculum builds on the student-teacher relationship and provides assignments and readings that highlight "negative capability" as opposed to offering definitive answers. The challenge is finding the balance between providing the conceptual scaffolding necessary for learning and growth to occur with the need to provide space for the student to negotiate their own answers.

Current Knowledge Base Including Psychological Theories

Dual MSW/MDiv students have learned a variety of psychological theories to assist them in understanding human behavior in the social environment. Two prominent theories that also offer corresponding modes of intervention are psychodynamic and cognitive-behavioral models. While psychological theories should not be used to deny or subvert beliefs in God, they can assist practitioners in understanding the role belief systems can play in clients' lives. For example, religion can function in a manner compatible with Winnicott's transitional phenomena as W.W. Meissner (2000) suggested, or represent clients' internal object relations as Rizutto (1979) proposed, or function in a role as powerful selfobject that repairs a fragmented self as Gay (1989) hypothesized. Likewise, religion can be understood as a cognitive schema (Koenig, 1995) or a worldview as Erikson asserted (Capps, 1998). A vital step in applying these understandings of religion is appreciating what the theories offer in terms of assessment. For example, suppose a clinician determines that a client has a religious understanding that is delusional in nature yet functions in a manner that organizes a chaotic internal world. After making this necessary psychological assessment that the clinician is trained to make, he or she can determine how to intervene in the client's world without challenging the belief system directly. If the clinician did not have an understanding of mental illness and the ways in which it can manifest, there may be a tendency to "correct" the client's "faulty" belief system as not being consistent with mainstream belief systems. In so doing, the client may become more agitated, disorganized, and ultimately flee treatment.

Critical Thinking

Utilizing psychological theories when appropriate is not recommended without understanding the limitations of these theories. In critiquing the psychological theories we study we look at several texts. A favorite text is edited by Spezzano and Gargiulo (1997) entitled "Soul on the Couch: Spirituality, Religion, and Morality in Contemporary Psychoanalysis." In his chapter, Rubin states: "The egocentric conception of 'I-ness' in psychoanalysis fosters a type of self-blindness and self-impoverishment. Thinking of the self as the center of the psychological and moral universe can foster a narrow and problematic way of seeing and relating to ourselves and others. . . . While every person may be at the center of his own world, no one is the center of the whole world. Thinking that we are–which individualism encourages–may compromise empathy and tolerance, foster disconnection from others, and engender self-alienation" (p. 85). Of course, it is important to retain psychological theories to understand that aspect of our clients that come "one at a time" but we must not forget the benefit from other belief systems that offer a window outside the narcissism of a separate self. For example, Rubin further discusses how the Buddhist practices of his analytic client enriched his own thinking about " . . . action, choice, moral commitment, and relational affiliations . . . " (p. 94). Rubin concludes that a psychoanalysis that is not only "self-centered might contribute to a civilization with less discontent" (p. 105). Moral questions pervade clinical work; unfortunately we are not always equipped to see these questions. Our curriculum does not attempt to answer these questions; rather, it highlights them and provides a space for students to examine them within the context of their own lives, the lives of their clients, and the lenses of their professions.

Postmodern Influences

What then can we offer the student in terms of conceptual scaffolding to guide their efforts to address these vital questions? Postmodernism is studied at this point in the course to fashion a broad enough umbrella to help clinicians in guiding their clients to find "meaning" in their personal narratives and spiritual beliefs. We examine "diverse ways of knowing" to appreciate feminist perspectives on spiritual narratives (Goldberger, Tarule, Clinchy, & Belenky, 1996). We look at the influence of trauma and the ways in which that shapes and colors a "quest for spirituality" (Barrett, 1999). And we learn how narrative theory can shape a style of practice that allows clients to "broaden their stories, rather than edit them" (Kelley in Northcut, 1999). Inherent in a discussion of why "meaning-making" is so essential to our lives and the lives of clients is an understanding of how neurobiology points us to the ways in which we are "hardwired" to make meaning in our lives as Ashbrook contemplated in his last book before he died (1997).

Postmodernism is not without its own failings in terms of a glorification of ambiguity that is not compatible with a spiritual narrative that should at least offer some comfort and ideas about meaning. However, postmodernism does diminish the needs of our respective professions to have the "truth" for all clients' problems. Rather it allows us to step back and make room to construct with clients their own "truth" within the context of their religious or spiritual tradition. Winnicott introduced the concept of transitional object and transitional space to reflect the need for a space between self and object that represents the twin realms of "neitherness" and "bothness" (Winnicott, 1971; Rothenberg, 1997). "Psychologically, this refers to the domain of experience that draws upon both self and other, but is neither occupied nor fully encompassed by either" (Rothenberg, 63). Our purpose is to model for the students a process of "space-making" for them to create within the therapeutic arena, yet also offers them space for their own development. By providing this space within a practice or methods course that is designed for students to integrate their beliefs and identities, students are free to develop an identity that is not limited to either social work or divinity, but can evolve into something unique, authentic and more meaningful to themselves and their clients.

CONCLUSION

There are no hard and fast rules for the formulation of a curriculum for students eager to find ways to integrate religion and spirituality in their clinical practice and in their professional identity. Every time this course is taught, the content necessarily "bends" in different directions to reflect current knowledge and the current needs of students. The curriculum must not be geared to provide dual degree students with a pre-formed integrated dual identity. Instead, we must try to nourish the "transitional space" necessary for "trying out" and discovering what that integration looks like for the individual student to draw from as they try to "meet the clients where they are." In true postmodern fashion, the integration of the MDiv and MSW identity lies in the dialogues students are able to construct with each other, their clients, and with their instructors.

REFERENCES

Anderson, H. (1999). Feet planted firmly in midair: A spirituality for family living. In F. Walsh (Ed.), *Spiritual resources in family therapy* (pp. 157-176). New York: Guilford Press.

Ashbrook, J.B., & Albright, C.R. (1997). A neurobiology of faith. *The humanizing brain: Where religion and neuroscience meet.* (pp. 3-28). Cleveland, Ohio: Pilgrim Press.

Barrett, M. J. (1999). Healing from trauma: The quest for spirituality. In F. Walsh (Ed.), *Spiritual resources in family therapy* (pp. 193-208). New York: Guilford Press.

Bate, W.J. (1963). *John Keats*. Cambridge, MA: Harvard University Press.

Belenky, M. F., Clinchy, B. M., Goldberger, N. R., & Tarule, J. M. (1986) *Women's ways of knowing: The development of self, voice, and mind.* New York: Basic Books.

Capps, W.H. (1998). Erik Erikson's contribution toward understanding religion. In R. S. Wallerstein & L. Goldberger (Eds.), *Ideas and identities: The life and work of Erik Erikson* (pp. 67-78). Matteson, CN: International Universities Press.

Case, P. W. (1997). Potential sources of countertransference among religious therapists. *Counseling and Values*, 41, 97-106.

Cornett, C. (1998). *The soul of psychotherapy*. New York: Free Press.

Fleischman, P. R. (1989). *The healing zone: Religious issues in psychotherapy*. New York: Parragon House.

Gay, V. (1989). *Understanding the occult: Fragmentation and repair of the self.* Minneapolis: Fortress.

Kelly, P. (1996). Narrative theory and social work treatment. In F. J. Turner (Ed.), *Social work treatment interlocking theoretical approaches, 4th Ed.* (pp. 461-479). New York: Free Press.

Koenig, H. G. (1995). Religion as cognitive schema. *The International Journal for the Psychology of Religion*, 5(1), 31-37.

Meissner, W. M. (2000). Psychoanalysis and religion: Current perspectives. In J. K. Boehnlein (Ed.), *Psychiatry and religion: The convergence of mind and spirit* (pp. 53-70). Washington, DC: American Psychological Association.

Pruyser, Paul (1977). The seamy side of religious beliefs. *Bulletin of the Menninger Clinic*, 41(4), 329-348.

Rizutto, A.-M. (1979). *The Birth of the Living God*. Chicago: University of Chicago.

Rothenberg, D. J. (1997). *Psychoanalysis and Jewish spirituality*. In C. Spezzano & C. Gargiulo (Eds.), *Soul on the couch: Spirituality religion & morality in contemporary psychoanalysis* 57-77, Hillsdale, NJ: Analytic Press.

Rubin, J. B. (1997). Psychoanalysis is self-centered. In C. Spezzano & C. Gargiulo (Eds.). *Soul on the couch: Spirituality religion & morality in contemporary psychoanalysis* 79-108. Hillsdale, NJ: Analytic Press.

Spezzano, C., & Gargiulo, G. J. (1997). *Soul on the couch: Spirituality, religion & morality in contemporary psychoanalysis*. Hillsdale, NJ: Analytic Press.

Walsh, F. (1999). *Spiritual resources in family therapy*. New York: Guilford Press.

Weingarten, K. (1999) Stretching to meet what's given: Opportunities for a spiritual practice. In F. Walsh (Ed.), *Spiritual resources in family therapy* (pp. 240-255). New York: Guilford Press.

Winnicott, D. W. (1971). *Playing and reality*. London: Tavistock.

Winnicott, D. W. (1971). *Through pediatrics to psychoanalysis*. New York: Basic Books.

The Diaconate as Dual-Skilled Ministry: A Proposal in Support of Dual Degree Programs for Formation

Margaret Ann Crain

SUMMARY. Since Vatican II, a number of Christian groups have sought to reclaim the diaconate in the service of the gospel. Roman Catholic deacons led the way in the United States but diaconal forms of ministry are now part of the structure in the Episcopal Church, the Evangelical Lutheran Church in America, and The United Methodist Church. Each ecclesiastical entity is still shaping formation programs appropriate to its form of diaconal ministry. This paper argues that the formation for deaconesses, diaconal ministers, and deacons who will seek to build compassionate communities must include skills in discernment that are learned through theological education *and* the tools for analysis, intervention and change that come from training in social work. The complexities of understanding systems and other factors that create oppression and the necessity of understanding deeply the call to "do justice, love mercy, and walk humbly with your God" (Micah 6:8) require creative approaches to forma-

---

Margaret Ann Crain, EdD, is an ordained Deacon in The United Methodist Church and Associate Professor of Christian Education and Director of Deacon Programs, Garrett-Evangelical Theological Seminary, 2121 Sheridan Road, Evanston, IL 60201 (E-mail: MargaretAnn.Crain@garrett.edu).

[Haworth co-indexing entry note]: "The Diaconate as Dual-Skilled Ministry: A Proposal in Support of Dual Programs for Formation." Crain, Margaret Ann. Co-published simultaneously in *Journal of Religion & Spirituality in Social Work: Social Thought* (The Haworth Social Work Practice Press, an imprint of The Haworth Press, Inc.) Vol. 24, No. 1/2, 2005, pp. 55-63; and: *Social Work and Divinity* (ed: Daniel Lee, and Robert O'Gorman) The Haworth Social Work Practice Press, an imprint of The Haworth Press, Inc., 2005, pp. 55-63. Single or multiple copies of this article are available for a fee from The Haworth Document Delivery Service [1-800-HAWORTH, 9:00 a.m. - 5:00 p.m. (EST). E-mail address: docdelivery@haworthpress. com].

http://www.haworthpress.com/web/JRSSW

Digital Object Identifier: 10.1300/J377v24n01_06

tion such as dual degree programs in social work and theology (MSW and MDiv). Dual degree programs can break down dualisms such as the "body/spirit" split. In order for this to work, the ecclesiastical bodies that supervise programs of formation and education must support candidates for the diaconate who need the dual degrees with money, time, and encouragement.

KEYWORDS. Diaconate, deacon, deaconess, formation, theological education, dual degree, social gospel, body/spirit dualism, master of divinity degree, master of social work degree

THE DIACONATE IN ITS CURRENT FORM

Several times a week the telephone rings in the deacon formation offices at our United Methodist seminary. At the other end is a person who is answering a call from God to "toil in the vineyard of compassion and justice." Sometimes the person has experienced a call to feed the hungry or house the homeless. Some speak of a call to minister to the needs of children and families engaged in custody struggles. Sometimes the person has heard the call to protect those most vulnerable in our society–children, the mentally ill, persons with HIV, those in the least skilled jobs, or those in the last stages of their lives. Always the person on the phone is seeking to respond to the great commandments for Christians: to love God and to love neighbor.

Diaconal ministry has re-emerged as a formal choice for Christians called to ministry in the last thirty years. Since Vatican II, a number of Christian churches have sought to reclaim the diaconate in the service of the gospel. Roman Catholic deacons led the way in the United States. Currently, ordained deacons may be found in the Episcopal Church, diaconal ministers in the Evangelical Lutheran Church in America, and ordained deacons in The United Methodist Church. In addition, deaconesses are associated with The United Methodist Church, Evangelical Lutheran Church in America, and others. Each ecclesiastical entity is still shaping formation programs appropriate for its form of the diaconate. This paper argues that the formation for deaconesses, diaconal ministers, and deacons who will seek to build compassionate communities must include skills in discernment that are learned through theological education *and* the tools for analysis, intervention and change that come from training in social work. For many in the diaconate, a dual degree is an appropriate choice for preparation and formation.

Presently, only a few formation programs for diaconal ministries require seminary education. The United Methodist Church and the Evangelical Lutheran Church in America have made graduate seminary level education a requirement. Other communions have developed formation and education programs separate from the seminaries, often administered by a diocese. The diaconate, emphasizing ministries of love and justice among the people and in the world, has attracted very diverse persons to diverse forms of service. Not all have the resources, both academic and financial, for graduate level academic seminary preparation. However, much of the work that deacons, deaconesses, and diaconal ministers do would be more effective and less vulnerable to actions that could lead to litigation if the diaconal minister were prepared both theologically and as a social worker.

Diaconal ministries were renewed in the modern Protestant world by the deaconess movement, primarily in the Methodist and Lutheran churches. Becoming a deaconess meant training for work of love and justice and becoming a part of a community, but it did not mean becoming cloistered or remaining celibate. "Of course, women's religious communities in the Roman Catholic Church had never ceased in their diaconal service." Led by Lucy Rider Meyer in the Chicago Training School for deaconesses, a Methodist institution that was eventually merged with Garrett Biblical Institute, the curriculum of these schools was balanced between theological studies (Bible, discipline and theology of the Methodist church, history of the Bible, church history) and women's leadership for social reform (lives of women reformers, world history, basic human anatomy and physiology, study of immigrant cultures and languages) (McConnell, 2003, pp. 36-38). The dual focus of social work and theological study, therefore, has been part of the formation of those called to and gifted for the diaconate for more than one hundred years.

Diaconal ministries in all their forms are pastoral, as they meet persons where they are and offer the spiritual resources for healing and wholeness that are part of the gospel of Jesus Christ. Learning to discern the will of God requires skills in theological reflection, a sure knowledge of the workings of the Church, a perspective on the past and present that comes from knowledge of church history and doctrine, skills in the practice of pastoral theology and Christian education, and thorough familiarity with the Bible. The Masters of Divinity degree offers these pastoral competencies.

The work of a deacon is also liturgical in most communions. The United Methodist deacon is to interrelate "worship in the gathered community with service to God in the world" (*Discipline*, 2000, par. 319), which is similar to the Roman Catholic deacon's "ministries of charity, liturgy, and the Word" (Shugrue, 1988, p. 188). In each of the ecumenical forms of the diaconate, the dual emphasis on church and world is stressed. Understanding the role of sacrament, in-depth knowledge of the Bible, and skills in theological reflection are critical for this sacramental, liturgical and teaching role. These skills are taught in a Masters of Divinity degree.

The work of a deacon is pastoral and liturgical, but also require the skills and knowledge that are developed in a graduate school of social work. Deacons (and the other forms of diaconal ministry) will work in congregations, institutions, and other settings where they provide services to persons who are hurting, either from actions of their own doing or from the oppression of systems. They will try to intervene on behalf of these human beings with the systems. They will try to help those persons to heal from the inside out and recover more healthy ways of dealing with the world and its problems. This paper will argue that the best training for persons whom God has called to the diaconate is a dual degree: Masters of Divinity and Masters of Social Work. The person on the telephone wants to know what options the seminary offers for an education that prepares her or him to do this ministry on behalf of the church but outside the walls of the church. These persons have heeded the call and answered, "Here I am!" They are looking for the professional tools and credentials for ministry that prepare them to address the social needs of those for whom they seek both compassion and justice. Both of these degrees attract people with strong desire to help other people.

Overcoming Dualisms

The diaconal calling that these persons have identified and to which they have responded mends the separation of social work from ministry. The theological imperative to love God and neighbor is integrated in diaconal work. These persons are called to bring healing to the world on behalf of the church. They are responding in faith to concrete injustices and needs. They do not see this call as groundbreaking. The way they envision answering their call may be groundbreaking or at least paradigm-challenging, however, because it breaks down the dualisms between clergy and laity, between church and world, between body and spirit, and between God's promise of new creation and the realities of oppressive structures that make living very difficult for many people in our society.

Pope John XXIII caught the essence of the diaconate and of social work when he told Loyola students, "The two most important things you possess are your minds and hearts. With one you learn, with the other, you love. I beg you to learn and love to your greatest capacity. The people in this world need all the love you and I can give them" (quoted on Loyola University Chicago web site, http://www.luc.edu/schools/socialwork/). The MSW degree prepares graduates to understand and diagnose human behavior so that they can lead more productive and functional lives. The clergy also are students of human behavior. Their work seeks to empower persons for fuller lives as Jesus says, "I came that they may have life and have it abundantly" (John 10:10, New Revised Standard Version). This is God's goal, shared by the professions of social work and ministry. The two professional degrees leading to these vocations have similar goals for graduates, but different content and different skills are taught. The combination of the two makes great sense for those who are called to a diaconal ministry that serves and loves the people of God. It may equally make sense for those who are called to the ministry of social work but do not practice it in formal relationship with a faith group.

However, the academic fields of social work and theology may not be hospitable to each other. They are very different disciplines, with little interaction in professional or scholarly discourse. A colleague of this writer at the seminary is said to have told students that the social sciences have nothing to teach about ministry. Theology, this colleague is reported to have said, is the only discipline to which we should look for truth and for guidance for the church.

This writer stands on the opposite side of that question. I believe that we must continue to seek the best of both disciplines as we seek to love the people in this world with all the love we can muster. Although I identify myself primarily as an ordained deacon of the United Methodist Church and I am a part of a seminary faculty, I call myself an ethnographic theologian. By that I mean that I study people, congregations, and cultures to learn about how God is acting in the world today and what God might be asking of us. I believe that we can indeed learn about who God is by listening to people of faith talk about how God has been present in their lives. We learn about God–that is, we do theology–by looking at the social interactions and structures that make up cultures. The study of the *ethnos* is a theological method. Therefore, my theology is the result of a combination of social science and theology. The social sciences are a part of the way that some of us in the seminary do our theological work.

We also, of course, learn about who God is by studying the rich heritage of the faith in the classical theological disciplines of Bible, Christian history, and historical and systematic theology. This theological method can operate independently of social science. To a great extent, this theological method dominates in academic schools of theology in the United States today.

Social sciences, however, give us the tools to see what IS as well as the tools to work toward what COULD BE. Social science has helped us to see how human beings are caught in webs of oppression that limit their possibilities. Social science has taught us how powerful identity is in shaping our lives. Social science has helped us to see how to help persons learn with varieties of intelligence as well as with many combinations of ability and disability. Social science has helped us to see the powerful influence of race and class and education. Social location is even more powerful in our human dance of life than is the proverbial "location, location, location" that determines the value of real estate. Thus, social science as it has developed into the profession of social work is a primary tool for theology and ministry, particularly as we seek to learn how to heal the wounded and make the world more faithful to God's will.

However, social science is not sufficient for the diaconate. Christian ministry must be evaluated by theological reflection. Keeping the work for compassion and justice in tune with God's ultimate will for creation is the work of theology. Studying the tradition, searching for the biblical witness with the best tools of exegesis, and considering what God wants for all people against concrete reality is the work of theological reflection. Toiling in the vineyard of compassion and justice requires the skills and resources of social sciences *and* the wisdom of theological reflection brought together in one person.

Social workers, those trained in the field of social work, who know how to bring resources and human need together, who provide the particular professional skills needed to effect change and to alleviate human misery, and who are also theologians are desperately needed. I want to suggest to you today that the diaconate is the church's affirmation of a ministry that combines social work and theology. An order of ministry with a dual focus on church and world and an orientation towards justice, the diaconate attempts to hold social work and theology in a single vision for ministry.

Yet, in each of its ecclesiological forms the deacon is struggling to articulate theologically its unique calling. Some point to the account in Acts where Stephen and others were set aside for the work of extending the table to those Hebrew and Greek widows who were in need. They were not officially called deacons but this passage does suggest that it is appropriate for the church to divide its functions and to set persons aside for specific tasks of a priestly or a diaconal nature.

A particularly apt phrase is: "[The diaconate] is the bond of living union between everyday Christian life and sacramental life that gives expression to and actualizes this union" (Kerkvoorde, p. 129). The author was talking about the work of deacons as leaders of the faith community participating in their concrete Christian life in this world. The deacon becomes a link between the sacramental and the everyday–a link located in the person of the deacon. The deacon functions "in all three areas of the Church's life: in the transmission of the Word, in the celebration of the sacraments, and in the community's active love" (Bishops, 1985, p. 14). The sacramental and the everyday are bound together in the body of the deacon who can only be ONE, not a split or dualistic being.

If the work of the deacon is to be located in two arenas–church and world–then the deacon needs to be trained for both places. As a representative of the church to the world and a leader of the church, the deacon "brings the poor to the church and the church to the poor." The Guidelines for formation of permanent deacons in the Catholic tradition revised in 1984 continue:

> The ancient tradition appears to indicate that it was because the deacon was the servant at the table of the poor that he had his distinctive liturgical roles of gathering the gifts and distributing communion at the Table of the Lord. . . . He thus symbolizes in his roles the grounding of the Church's life in the Eucharist and the mission of the Church in the loving service of the needy. (Bishops, 1985, p. 15).

In the complex cultural and social world wherein the church has its mission, a deacon must be highly trained in order to ascertain the systems and structures that limit and oppress the people whom we are called to love. "This ministry of love is also a ministry of justice that aims not only at meeting immediate needs but also at addressing their structural and institutional causes" (Bishops, 1985, p. 18). Social workers, those trained in the field of social work, who know how to bring resources to human need, are equipped to serve "at the table of the poor." Theologians are equipped to serve at the "Table of the Lord."

The Evangelical Lutheran Church in American articulates a similar dual focus for its diaconal ministers. They are "rooted in the Word of God" and "trained to carry out a particular service" (The Evangelical Lutheran Church in America, p. E-1). Diaconal ministers are also to "give particular attention to ministries at the boundaries between church and world" and to "exemplify the life of Christ-like service addressing all forms of human need."

The United Methodist 2000 *Discipline* proclaims that the ministry of the ordained deacon "exemplifies and leads the Church in the servanthood every Christian is called to live both in the church and in the world. The deacon embodies the interrelationship between worship in the gathered community and service to God in the world" (par. 310). With co-author Jack Seymour, this writer contends that "the heart of a deacon, the heart of service, is extended into all the world through the love of God and the ministries of the Church" (Crain, p. 145). This diaconal ministry on behalf of the embodied people of God becomes a sign of God's love even though it requires the skills of the profession of social work. The theologically trained social worker understands that she or he has the resources to offer hope beyond what the agency or institution can offer. God's grace works together with programs and funds to effect healing in people's minds, bodies, and spirits.

Hence we come to the rationale for dual degree programs in theology and social work. Those who are called to the diaconal ministries face a complex world and a church whose voice of authority has dimmed. The clergy is besmirched by scandal and plagued with ineffectiveness. Violence rules the street and invades our homes. The poor get poorer and the middle class are paralyzed by fears of stock market crashes and the possibility of being "downsized." The task of building compassionate communities in the midst of these intractable and complex tensions is not for the fainthearted or poorly trained. Our deacons and diaconal ministers who will seek to build compassionate communities need all the discernment that a theological education provides and the tools for change that come from training in social work.

Practical Implications of Dual Degree Programs

The notion of a dual degree may seem ridiculously idealistic. It takes a long time–probably five years. It costs a great deal in both time and money–five years of full time schooling. Even a credentialed person in full time ministry will never be paid a large salary. The debt load from graduate school will be huge. The urgent needs of vulnerable people seem to outweigh the value of graduate professional study. Justifying five or six years of expensive graduate education becomes difficult in light of the persons who are hurting and needing help today! Answering God's call to toil in the vineyard of compassion and justice may not seem consistent with the need for credentials and professional training.

Therefore, the committees and hierarchies of the Christian communities that oversee the education and formation of persons called to the diaconate should support dual degree programs in theology and social work. Support means to explain why both sets of skills are crucial. Support means financial assistance. Support means patience as persons prepare themselves for the work that makes the gospel incarnate in the realities of life. A combination of theology and social work will provide leaders for the mission of Christ to love our neighbor both within the church and within the world in the 21st century.

REFERENCES

Bishop's Committee on the Permanent Diaconate, National Conference of Catholic Bishops (1985). *Permanent deacons in the United States: Guidelines on their formation and ministry.*

Book of discipline of the United Methodist Church 2000. Nashville, TN: United Methodist Publishing House

Crain, M. A., & Seymour, J. L. (2001). *The heart of a deacon: The new United Methodist diaconate.* Nashville TN: Abingdon Press.

Kerkvoorde, OSB, D. A. "The theology of the diaconate," p. 129 in Bishops' Committee on the Permanent Diaconate, National Conference of Catholic Bishops (no date), *Foundations for the Renewal of the Diaconate.*

McConnell, S. (February 2003). *Canadian deaconess and missionary education for women training to live the social gospel: The Methodist national training school and the Presbyterian deaconess and missionary training home, 1893-1926.* Unpublished thesis, University of Winnipeg.

Shugrue, T. J. (1988). *Service ministry of the deacon: Bishop's committee on the permanent diaconate.* Washington DC: National Conference of Catholic Bishops.

The Evangelical Lutheran Church in America (no date). "Candidates for Diaconal Ministry" *Candidacy manual: Division of ministry of The Evangelical Lutheran Church in America.* Chicago, Illinois, p. E-1.

Collaborative Responses to the Demands of Emerging Human Needs: The Role of Faith and Spirituality in Education for Social Work

Edwin M. Conway

SUMMARY. The paper explores the disintegration and integration which exist between faith and religion and social work and learning. There is a brief explanation of Catholic Papal Teachings and Catholic Social Teaching as a demonstration of *de facto* concordance between social work and religion. The paper contains citations based on the current social principles of the Catholic Church, several recent papal exhortations and encyclicals. These readings highlight the need for good social work practice. The paper ends with some practical suggestions in ways to promote collaboration between the two fields of endeavor. *[Article copies available for a fee from The Haworth Document Delivery Service: 1-800-HAWORTH. E-mail address: <docdelivery@haworthpress.com> Website: <http://www.HaworthPress.com> © 2005 by The Haworth Press, Inc. All rights reserved.]*

Most Reverend Edwin M. Conway, DD, was Auxiliary Bishop of the Roman Catholic Archdiocese of Chicago, IL, a Member of Catholic Health Association Sponsor committee, and National Episcopal Advisor to Diocesan Coordinators of Health Care.

The author died on August 9, 2004.

[Haworth co-indexing entry note]: "Collaborative Responses to the Demands of Emerging Human Needs: The Role of Faith and Spirituality in Education for Social Work." Conway, Edwin M. Co-published simultaneously in *Journal of Religion & Spirituality in Social Work: Social Thought* (The Haworth Social Work Practice Press, an imprint of The Haworth Press, Inc.) Vol. 24, No. 1/2, 2005, pp. 65-77; and: *Social Work and Divinity* (ed: Daniel Lee, and Robert O'Gorman) The Haworth Social Work Practice Press, an imprint of The Haworth Press, Inc., 2005, pp. 65-77. Single or multiple copies of this article are available for a fee from The Haworth Document Delivery Service [1-800-HAWORTH, 9:00 a.m. - 5:00 p.m. (EST). E-mail address: docdelivery@haworthpress.com].

http://www.haworthpress.com/web/JRSSW

Digital Object Identifier: 10.1300/J377v24n01_07

KEYWORDS. Catholic social teaching, faith and social work, church and social work

Society is crying out in need for remedies that are provided by both fields of study, divinity and social work. It is a blessing that in some institutions they can be combined in the same path of studies, forming a practitioner who can bring an integrated wealth of goodness to the people they serve. I will focus on the integration of faith and social work from a Catholic point of view.

Weavings, a quarterly publication, attempts to gather the thinking and reflections on a focused and specific element of spiritual development in the Christian life. Each issue features articles by Catholic, Protestant, Orthodox and other Christian writers. The fall 2001 issue had the theme of "The Road." One of the articles is entitled "A Knight of the Road" (Clarke, 2001). It deals with the life of Ignatius of Loyola, the founder of the Society of Jesus, the Jesuits, the religious sponsors of Loyola University. The author traced three phases in the life of Ignatius as he made his way from conversion through ministry.

The first phase was solitude. Ignatius found himself the great sinner, and after hermitic prayer and separation, he discovered the beginnings of hope in God's mercy. The journey was far from complete. He next realized that he was called to share both his sinfulness and newly found forgiveness with others. This sharing was not only a support for him but also means of his recognition that the Christian life is developed in and with the Church, not in an individualistic stance. Hence Ignatius gathered to himself like spirited people who were aware of these same grace filled gifts. Lastly, as he was growing in his awareness of his union with God, Ignatius came to realize that the Christian is also called to be engaged with the world. So, through the gifts of grace and insight, he and his band of acquaintances committed themselves to one another in the service of the Church, in the form of the Society of Jesus. His journey of development had now become firmly fixed on a continuing path and journey of engagement and collaboration with others.

As I reflect over the "Road" article, I think of the fact that as people of faith we often talk not only of our Christian life being a journey, but we also realize that this journey requires us to integrate all of life's encounters into that path of development. That task of integration is never ended. We long for it to end, to be settled, to be stilled, but it will not respond to our expectations. As with Ignatius, we think we have come to a fixed point, only to find out once again that we are being beckoned onward to a new level of engagement, involvement and integration.

So it is with the life of faith and the profession of social work. There is much that these two ways have in common. To be realistic, however, the possibility of discord and dysfunction between the two fields and within the person can also easily arise, if misunderstanding and misinterpretation take over.

I will deal with common areas of goals and knowledge first.

I. Integration

Faith and social work on the level of truth should not have any struggle or conflict. As truth they both share a common gift from God and a common goal. Seeking and striving after truth can provide an opening and blossoming of the human person to further and deeper development of the fullness of life. In recent years Pope John Paul II has published an encyclical letter *Fides et Ratio*, *Faith and Reason* (1998), which deals with the integration and reconciliation between faith, reason, science and knowledge.

> Both the light of reason and the light of faith come from God, he [St. Thomas Aquinas, *Contra Gentiles*, I, 7] argued; hence there can be no contradiction between them. (John Paul II, 1998, #43, p. 65)

> The key point and almost the kernel of the solution which, with all the brilliance of his prophetic intuition, he [Aquinas] gave to the new encounter of faith and reason was a reconciliation between the secularity of the world and the radicality of the Gospel, thus avoiding the unnatural tendency to negate the world and its values, while at the same time keeping faith with the supreme and inexorable demands of the supernatural order. (John Paul II, 1998, #43, p. 66)

> Deprived of what Revelation offers, reason has taken sidetracks which expose it to the danger of losing sight of its final goal. Deprived of reason, faith has stressed feeling and experience, and so runs the risk of no longer being a universal proposition. (John Paul II, 1998, #48, p. 73)

> There is thus no reason for competition of any kind between reason and faith: each contains the other, and has its own scope for action. (John Paul II, 1998, #17, p. 29)

The Catechism of the Catholic Church is the day-to-day instructional document that brings the spirit of the Second Vatican Council into Catholics' lives. It clearly calls upon the devotee to be about the search for truth in the pursuit of accepting God's love and creation in the everyday elements of life.

> Believing is possible only by grace and the interior helps of the Holy Spirit. But it is no less true that believing is an authentically human act. Trusting in God and cleaving to the truths He has revealed are contrary neither to human freedom nor to human reason. (1994 et seq., #154, p. 42)

> Consequently, methodical research in all branches of knowledge, provided it is carried out in a truly scientific manner and does not override moral laws, can never conflict with the faith, because the things of the world and the things of faith derive from the same God. (1994 et seq., #159, p. 43)

Social Work is an asset for the people with whom I work, as any dually trained person could attest. The discipline that flows from the training that a skilled practitioner has received allows them to listen with an empathetic and discerning ear. The dually trained worker can analyze and integrate the communication of the parishioner or the client in a way that leads to the ability to make the appropriate and integrated response, freeing the person to be open to and embracing further development.

The dually trained clinician can more perceptively enter the life of the client to recognize and assist the client in discerning what is arising from spiritual development, in distinction to psychological experiences.

Sorting out the elements of one's life that interfere with spiritual growth is not easy. The skills provided by the integration of social work afford the opportunity to classify, delineate and address in a productive way human responses to situations and failings. The client with a developed spiritual life or striving toward that development, can benefit from such a trained worker. It is a blessing to be engaged with a worker who can readily understand the human struggle in light of belief in divinely nurtured elements of life.

In my own *personal* faith life I have found the study, the practice and the integration of social work to be a benefit. The spiritual writers of the Church recall that prayer is the raising of the hearts and minds to God in an integrated offering of the whole person. Often persons spend the majority of time in prayer, however, dealing only with the mental aspects of their lives. To concentrate on the emotional needs and responses in prayer is much more demanding and telling. The discipline of social work as I have experienced it has been an asset in the development of a prayer life, which is spiritually formational.

II. Disintegration

We know of points in history (and the present) in which there has been disintegration if not hostility between the fields of social work and religion. This breakdown has arisen when the goals, expertise and limitations of each field are not understood or accepted.

The field of religion, faith, and spirituality has its origins in God. Thus faith is a gift. It is a mystery, which one cannot fully fathom. Theologians describe it an act of infinite unconditional love on God's part to bring us into existence and sustain us in life (McBrian,1981, p. 38). The other side of spirituality and religion deals with the human response to the revelation of God's love. This reality cannot be subjected to the limits or discipline of the scientific method. As persons composed of both body and soul, that integrated reality cannot be ignored. We have only to look to the research being conducted on the effects of pastoral services in hospitals and the state of recuperation to see the effect of one area on the other (Dossey, 1993). The attempts to dichotomize the human person have left us on one hand with Nihilism and on the other with Jansenism.

The dealing with sin or the specific and appropriate guilt that arises from sinning is beyond the scope of the field of social work. So often the breakdown between social work, psychology, and the helping professions and religion occurs because of the disagreement over what is appropriate guilt and its remedy. When the practitioner attempts to substitute the therapeutic relationship for the expression of repentance and God's forgiving love, the harmony between social work and faith break down.

When the attempt is made to merely view and work with the client as a material body and not a person of spirit, then disintegration sets in. The same destructive phenomenon occurs when the limits of the therapeutic intervention fail to acknowledge that the person may be troubled by a reality beyond the scope of social work, either totally or partially. The questions of heaven, afterlife, grace and discipleship are just a few of the elements that may fall outside the limitations of social work.

Religion and faith deny full goodness to the person when they fail to appreciate that the person may have a distorted psychological image of

God or an inordinately developed sense of guilt which will not allow him or her to be open to the prompting of the Spirit. At other times the minister may not be aware of the need to recognize the assistance that social work can be to the person to correctly orient them to spiritual direction. For instance, difficulty can arise where the religious counselor doesn't recognize the presence of pathological guilt, and thus long-term harm can come to the counselee or penitent.

Sometimes the religious leader will not be sufficiently aware of the delicate balance of human nature and grace in the life of his/her parishioner. This balance of recognizing the beauty of God's creation and the mystery of His grace has plagued the Christian and the Church from its foundation. There seems to be a tendency to slide totally toward one direction as opposed to the other. The destruction of this balance is reflected in many of the schisms and the heresies that pepper the history of the church. Pelagianism asserted that our works gained God's grace (McBrien, 1995, p. 981). Manichaeism taught that the disciple should abstain from all contact with the material (McBrien, 1995, p. 810). Gnosticism held that a few of the elect had a special singular knowledge of the Lord (McBrien, 1995, p. 563). Donatism pushed us to an inordinate rigid standard of holiness disregarding the reality of human nature. (McBrien, 1995, p. 431) The "ism's" go on in each generation as we seek to balance the wholesomeness of the human person and God's freely given grace.

Members of the Church at times have lapsed into Fideism (McBrien, 1995, p. 509). Fideism denies the possibility of arriving at certain knowledge of the existence of God and the facts of revelation by natural powers. The followers of Fideism think that the only source of moral and religious knowledge lies exclusively in divine revelation.

While it is a matter of creed that Church is of divine origin and continuous nurturing, it also is human in its relationships and life. This human element can become unbalanced in the use of power, judgement making, inappropriate teaching and preaching and in the exercise of control. Failure to consistently return to the realization of the needs that arise in any human structuring, in relationships, especially those that are hierarchical, and in an ambiance that is filled with ceremony and mystery can be destructive of the person and their spiritual development.

In the pastoral life of the Church, too often the generous expression of faith catapults one into service of their brothers and sisters. This reaching out to help is often done without realizing the inappropriateness of the response to the person in need or acknowledging the assistance that professional training could give to better handle the situation.

III. Integration Based Upon a Theology of Social Doctrine

There is a natural integration between spirituality and social work. The tradition of the Church strongly teaches that we are clearly called to care for one another. The Catholic tradition flows from the very central doctrine of the Church, teaching that God is Father and creatures are therefore brother and sister to one another. They imitate the God who made them, a God of love: "Father, Son, and Holy Spirit." This central reality is spelled out clearly in what is called the Social Tradition and Social Teachings of the Church. Father William Byron (1999), the former president of Catholic University of America reflects on the 1998 Catholic Bishops' Statement, *Sharing Catholic Social Teaching: Challenges and Directions–Reflections of the U. S. Bishops*:

The Principle of Human Dignity

> Every human being is created in the image of God and redeemed by Jesus Christ, and therefore is invaluable and worthy of respect as a member of the human family.

The Principle of Respect for Human Life

> Every person, from the moment of conception to natural death, has inherent dignity and a right to life consistent with that dignity.

The Principle of Association

> Our tradition proclaims that the person is not only sacred but also special. How we organize our society–in economics and politics, in law and policy–directly affects human dignity and the capacity of individuals to grow in community.

The Principle of Participation

> We believe people have the right and a duty to participate in society, seeking together the common good and well being of all, especially the poor and vulnerable.

The Principle of Preferential Protection for the Poor and Vulnerable

> In a society marred by deepening divisions between rich and poor, our tradition recalls the story of the Last Judgment (Mt 25:32-46) and instructs us to put the needs of the poor and vulnerable first.

The Principle of Solidarity

> Catholic Social Teaching proclaims that we are our brothers' and sisters' keepers, wherever they live. We are one human family. . . . Learning to practice the virtue of solidarity means learning that 'loving our neighbor' has global dimensions in an interdependent world.

The Principle of Stewardship

> The Catholic tradition insists that we show our respect for the Creator by our stewardship of creation.

The Principle of Subsidiarity

> [Here is defined] responsibilities and limits of government, and the essential roles of voluntary associations.

The Principle of Human Equality

> Equality of all persons comes from their essential dignity. . . . While differences in talents are a part of God's plan, social and cultural discrimination in fundamental rights . . . are not compatible with God's design.

The Principle of the Common Good

> The common good is understood as the social conditions that allow people to reach their full human potential and realize their human dignity.

The United States Catholic Bishops issued this reflection, as they have in many similar variations, because there is a sense that a newer generation of Catholics has lost the understanding of our social awareness and traditions. The Bishops have asked that Catholic educational institutions from elementary schools through the university level begin to teach once again the Social Tradition of the Church. In fact, the Vatican currently, at the request of Pope John Paul II, is publishing a special catechism on Catholic Social Teaching to help focus the present generation's responsibilities on the needs and resources of society (*The Social Agenda of the Catholic Church*, 2002). These initiatives will provide a practical coupling of religion and social work.

One can also learn of the social teachings, especially the *common good*, in a quite useful and down-to-earth way by listening to some of the practical insights the present Pope, John Paul II, has given in the Apostolic Exhortation *Ecclesia in America, The Church in America* (1999). This letter flowed from the deliberations and discussions of the Synod on the Americas, November 1997. Representative Bishops and experts met for a month surfacing the strengths and weaknesses of the nations of this hemisphere in relationship to the Church. The Apostolic Exhortation, *Ecclesia in America*, is not only a summary of findings but a call to face our bond as a people who have a dynamic effect on one another. While we are very diverse nations in this hemisphere, we also have many areas of relationship that can be a resource or a detriment for one another. The effects of our Social Teachings extend not only through the streets of my neighborhood or city, region or country; but also are called for in our international relationships. Here are a few verbatim quotes from the document.

- The phenomenon of urbanization [therefore] presents great challenges for the Church's pastoral action, which must address cultural rootlessness, loss of family traditions and of the people's particular religious traditions. As a result, faith is often weakened because it is deprived of the expressions that helped to keep it alive.
- A feature of the contemporary world is the tendency towards globalization, a phenomenon which, although not exclusively American, is more obvious and has greater repercussions in America.
- The Synod Fathers voiced concern about the external debt afflicting many American nations and expressed solidarity with them.
- Corruption [in private life and public life] is often among the causes of crushing public debt, and is therefore a problem, which needs to be considered carefully.
- The drug trade and drug use represents a grave threat to the social fabric of American nations. The drug trade contributes to crime and violence, to the destruction of family life, to the physical and

emotional destruction of many individuals and communities, especially among the young.
- To men and women, the crown of the entire process of creation, the Creator entrusts the care of the earth. This brings concrete obligations in the area of ecology for every person. Fulfillment of these obligations supposes an openness to a spiritual and ethical perspective capable of overcoming selfish attitudes and life-styles which lead to the depletion of natural resources (John Paul II, 1999, #56ff. 17).

These verbatim snippets from the document call to be about conscious efforts to seek what is wholesome and beneficial for sisters and brothers everywhere. To some they may not appear to be the subject matter of spirituality or religion. The point of the Apostolic Exhortation is just that, through service of others we deepen relationship to God. The Synod participants and the Pope ask urge to look more deeply and sharply to see what mutual role one may play in the lives and relationships of sisters and brothers at home as well as in other parts of the hemisphere. One trained in both social work and theology can play a unique and productive role in bringing the resources of the Church and the community to address these and other issues in the world. Everything in the field of social work and in the Church challenges us to bring others and ourselves to confront these dysfunctional elements in our communities. Far from allowing an artificial barrier between social work and faith to arise, the most realistic and helpful way to bring assistance to these issues and many more is by using the resources of both entities.

IV. Some Practical Suggestions

The Social Tradition of the Church and the practice of social work can be wedded in an alliance to better the community and aid the individual. Here are suggestions that may stimulate more profound thinking on the development of the dual degree program.

A. Continue to highlight the dual degree program. The marketing for this sequence should also be done in church settings to bring awareness of the program to the pastoral life of the Church.
B. Do not shy away from the reality that many young people today are challenging society and its institutions on the role of spirituality in their lives. While the pursuit of spirituality may not as yet have been

fashioned into a structured religion or institutional church, to ignore the reality seems not to face the needs of the emerging students.

C. In line with the spiritual search of the student today, schools of social work could make available a list of consultants, spiritual advisors, and formators to assist the student in that journey.

D. There is a rich heritage and base of literature in the Catholic Church as well as other ecclesial bodies dealing with social doctrine. It may be meritorious if the schools of social work looked toward establishing a sequence of studies around this literature. This could be followed with a practicum in ecclesial settings that would programmatically integrate the theoretical learning.

E. Design opportunities for academic leadership to explore *Sharing Catholic Social Teaching: Challenges and Directions–Reflections of the U.S. Bishops* (1998) and similar Church statements that encourage and challenge the teaching of social principles in our institutions of higher learning.

F. Explore the possibilities that lie within a relationship with other departments and schools in the university to respond to the expressed need of the students or communities for exposure to the theology of social principals and pastoral practice. For instance there is an obvious call for ethical training in our business education as well as in the healing professions.

G. Seize the opportunities to engage with churches in sharing the wholesomeness that good social work practice can bring to the life of the Church. This relationship can especially be forged in the institutional settings at the local level and national level. Many faith-based social service entities already have established these ecumenical and inter-faith relationships. It would be a boon to fulfilling their goals if schools of social work would join with them.

H. There are hundreds of thousands of paraprofessionals laboring in our parishes and ecclesial institutions. They and their directors are in need of quality and appropriate instruction to both support and delineate the limits of their service. With a few exceptions, schools of social work have been slow to enter into a relationship with these agencies and entities to supply this education. It could be a fruitful field of endeavor.

I. There are numerous meetings requiring facilitators, which occur under ecclesial auspices each day. There are multiple boards, which require experienced participants at every level of Church life. There are continuous repetitious neuralgic situations within the Church, which require negotiated solutions and/or healing.

> The appropriate dually trained worker could be a great asset in these settings.

I have been involved in administration and social service delivery as well as pastoral ministry for over forty years. None of these suggestions can be realized without financial support and people to participate in the programs. It is difficult to have a mission without a market and margin. On the other hand, if we do not begin to discuss and design responses to the needs we are experiencing, we will continue to become less effective as church and educational enterprises in peoples' lives.

In conclusion, I return to quoting the concluding thoughts of Pope John Paul II in his encyclical *Sollicitudo Rei Socialis* (1987). The words help us to realize how clearly the pastoral life of the Church is practically wedded to the service of people.

> I wish to *appeal* with simplicity and humility to *everyone*, to all men and women without exception. I wish to ask them to be convinced of the seriousness of the present moment and of each one's responsibility, and to implement–by the way they live as individuals and as families, by the use of their resources, by their civic activity, by contributing to economic and political decisions and by personal commitment to national and international undertakings–the *measures* inspired by solidarity and love of preference for the poor. This is what is demanded by the present moment and above all by the very dignity of the human person, the indestructible image of God and the creator, which is *identical* in each of us. In this commitment, the sons and daughters of the Church must serve as examples and guides, for they are called upon, in conformity with the programme announced by Jesus himself in the synagogue at Nazareth, to "preach good news to the poor . . . to proclaim release to the captives and recovering of sight to the blind, to set at liberty those who are oppressed, to proclaim the acceptable year of the Lord." (Lk 4: 18-19) (John Paul II, 1987, #47)

REFERENCES

Byron, W. (1999). Building Blocks, *Charities USA*, Second Quarter.

Catechism of the Catholic Church (1994 et seq.). Washington, DC: United States Conference of Catholic Bishops.

Clarke, T. (2001). A Knight of the Road, *Weavings*, November December, Vol. 16, No. 6.

Dossey, L. (1993). *Healing Words: The Power of Prayer and Practice of Medicine*, San Francisco: Harper.

John Paul II (1987). *Sollicitudo Rei Socialis*, Washington, DC: United States Conference of Catholic Bishops.

John Paul II (1998). *Fides et Ratio*. Washington, DC: United States Conference of Catholic Bishops.

John Paul II (1999). *Ecclesia in America*, Washington, DC: U.S. Conference of Catholic Bishops.

McBrien, R. P. (1981). *Catholicism (Study Edition)*. Minneapolis: Winston Press.

McBrien, R. P. (1995). *The Harper-Collins Encyclopedia of Catholicism* (1995). New York: HarperCollins Publisher.

Sirico, R. A., and Zieba M., OP. (Eds.) (2002). *The Social Agenda of the Catholic Church: The Magisterial Texts*, New York: Burns and Oates, Continuum International Publishing Group.

United States Catholic Bishops (1998). *Sharing Catholic Social Teaching: Challenges and Directions–Reflections of the U.S. Bishops*, Washington, DC: United States. Conference of Catholic Bishops.

Integrating Religion and Social Work in Dual Degree Programs

Edward R. Canda

SUMMARY. This article offers challenges, suggestions and examples for integrating insights from religion and social work in the context of masters level dual degree programs that link social work and other fields of study about religion, such as theology, pastoral counseling, and religious studies. The author first relates some personal and professional experiences regarding his own journey during the past 30 years in trying to find ways to connect religious studies, pastoral counseling, and social work. Next, the article presents suggestions for mutually beneficial ways that fields for studying religion and social work can challenge each other. Finally, several practical suggestions are given for designing integrated religion and social work dual degree programs. *[Article copies available for a fee from The Haworth Document Delivery Service: 1-800-HAWORTH. E-mail address: <docdelivery@haworthpress.com> Website: <http://www.HaworthPress.com> © 2005 by The Haworth Press, Inc. All rights reserved.]*

Edward R. Canda, PhD, is Professor and Chair of the PhD Program in Social Work, as well as Courtesy Professor of Religious Studies, University of Kansas. He has Masters degrees in Religious Studies and Social Work and a PhD in Social Work.

Address correspondence to: Edward R. Canda, PhD, School of Social Welfare, The University of Kansas, 1545 Lilac Lane, Lawrence, KS 66044-3184 (E-mail: edc@ku.edu or www.socwel.ku.edu/canda).

[Haworth co-indexing entry note]: "Integrating Religion and Social Work in Dual Degree Programs." Canda, Edward R. Co-published simultaneously in *Journal of Religion & Spirituality in Social Work: Social Thought* (The Haworth Social Work Practice Press, an imprint of The Haworth Press, Inc.) Vol. 24, No. 1/2, 2005, pp. 79-91; and: *Social Work and Divinity* (ed: Daniel Lee, and Robert O'Gorman) The Haworth Social Work Practice Press, an imprint of The Haworth Press, Inc., 2005, pp. 79-91. Single or multiple copies of this article are available for a fee from The Haworth Document Delivery Service [1-800-HAWORTH, 9:00 a.m. - 5:00 p.m. (EST). E-mail address: docdelivery@haworthpress.com].

http://www.haworthpress.com/web/JRSSW

Digital Object Identifier: 10.1300/J377v24n01_08

KEYWORDS. Religion, religious studies, spirituality, social work, education

INTRODUCTION

This article offers challenges, suggestions and examples for integrating insights from religion and social work in the context of masters level dual degree programs that link social work and other fields of study about religion, such as religious studies, theology, pastoral counseling, ministry, Jewish Studies, and Buddhist Studies. It presents reflections on the author's experiences during the past 30 years in trying to find ways to connect religious studies, pastoral counseling, and social work. It considers some beneficial challenges that studies of religion and social work can offer each other when they are connected in dual degree programs. Finally several practical suggestions are given for designing integrated religion and social work dual degree programs. These suggestions are shaped by the author's standpoint as a social work professor with a strong commitment to the field of academic religious studies and the hope that these tentative ideas will encourage continued dialogue about ways to connect studies of religion and social work in university education. In order to convey a sense of realism, self-reflections by the author will be presented in first person narrative style.

A CIRCUITOUS PATH INTO RELIGIOUS STUDIES AND SOCIAL WORK

I have had an interest in both religion and social service from a very early age. My Catholic upbringing in a devout family and Catholic school system instilled in me an appreciation for both the contemplative and socially engaged aspects of spirituality. By the time of high school, I was exploring both comparative religions and social service volunteerism and activism. As an undergraduate student at Kent State University, I majored in anthropology, focusing on East Asian cultures and religions. Then, I was very fortunate to become a Fulbright Graduate Fellow of East Asian philosophy in South Korea.

However, my peregrinations were not finished. After much soul searching, I decided to complete an MA degree in Religious Studies at the University of Denver. Religious Studies is an academic field dedicated to the scholarly study of diverse religious traditions, including their histories, beliefs, practices, and places within their cultural contexts (Capps, 1995). While completing that degree, along with courses at Iliff School of Theology, I tremendously enjoyed the academic study of religions. But I also felt that something was missing for me. The various religious traditions I studied all examined the nature and causes of suffering in the human condition. They all prescribed various remedies. But while I could study this, I did not know how to actually apply the insights to help people directly.

Some vocational counseling helped me sort out the obvious–that through my 25 years up to that time, I had felt two distinct callings: one to the study of religion and the other to the doing of service. Unfortunately, I did not have a clear design about how to link social service and religious studies. I did not have any career guidance, teachers, or role models who could help me work out the connections. Rather, I followed my intuitions and interests as these two kinds of pursuits wound through each other. I had to figure out how to put them together on my own. At that point, I decided that I needed to study professional social work. This brought me to The Ohio State University in 1980, where I was fortunate to meet faculty who encouraged my efforts to begin integrating the two callings into one vocation and professional role.

During my MSW and doctoral studies in social work, I applied my interests in the cross-cultural study of religion to social work by continuing studies in psychological anthropology and religious perspectives on social work and by teaching comparative religious studies courses. As a social work student and practitioner, I worked mostly with Southeast Asian refugees and people dealing with cross-cultural transition and relationships. These practice situations gave opportunities for me to apply insights from anthropology and religious studies to social work.

However, during that time, 1980-1986, I found a perplexing situation in the profession of social work regarding the lack of integration of spirituality. I learned that the profession originated with strong influences from Christian and Jewish traditions and institutions of service. I developed great appreciation of the field's commitment to values and purposes to alleviate suffering and to promote justice, so that people could achieve their fullest potential. The social work theoretical base emphasized how important it is to understand and relate to people as whole beings in their social contexts. These commitments to service and holistic understanding seemed very familiar to me from my studies of religions, as though professional social work had become a kind of secular religion. However, as Siporin (1985 & 1986) pointed out, social work education and scholarly writing at the time typically neglected or even ostracized the spiritual aspect of people. I wondered, "How can a profession with religious origins, sharing aspirations with the best aspects of religions, and claiming to deal with the whole person, cut off the spiritual realm of life?"

I was in a quandary. Having pursued religious studies, I found great insights into spirituality, but little help in how to apply them to service. Having pursued social work, I found great insights into human service, but little help in how to do this in a spiritually sensitive manner. The challenge before me was to find how to connect these two kinds of insights. The gap between social work and spirituality was a serious problem, not only for myself, but also for the profession of social work as a whole. In order for social work to fulfill its own promise, it would need to reincorporate the spiritual dimension. For this reason, I decided to make that the central question of my doctoral dissertation work. Thus, I was able to find about 20 other scholars around the country who shared this concern and who offered many insights and suggestions (Canda, 1988a & 1988b).

Eventually, this networking enabled me to create the Society for Spirituality and Social Work in 1990. As many educators and practitioners connected, our synergy built up momentum for spiritually sensitive social work. As one indicator of this change, the number of MSW programs around the country offering courses on religion and spirituality changed from approximately 4 in 1986 to around 75 today (Russel, 1998 and personal communication). Most of these developed in the past 8 years. There are also about 25 cooperative graduate educational programs between social work and theology, ministry, pastoral care, Jewish studies, or religious studies (Simpkinson, Wengell, & Casavant, 1994). Now, there is so much productive activity in research, teaching, conferences, practice, and publications related to religion and spirituality that it is difficult to keep up with it (e.g., Bullis, 1996; Canda & Furman, 1999; Canda, Nakashima, Burgess, Russel, & Barfield, 2003; Cnaan, 1999; Ellor, Netting, & Thibault, 1999; Van Hook, Hugen, & Aguilar, 2002).

The good news from all of this is that now social work students have the opportunity and encouragement in many social work programs to connect spirituality with social work. It is no longer necessary for students to follow such a long circuitous path as I in order to find the junction between religion and social work.

However, integration between religious perspectives and professional social work poses challenges related to differing concerns and assumptions between them. Of course, there are vast differences between religions so it is difficult to make generalizations about 'religion' or 'a religious perspective.' There is also a great variety in types and contexts of social work theory and practice. So the following discussion makes broad comparisons with caution only for the sake of encouraging discussion.

CONTRASTS AND CHALLENGES BETWEEN RELIGION AND SOCIAL WORK

First, in a very broad way, one can say that religions claim to have a grasp of ultimate truth, or at least truths that come from sacred sources of inspiration and theological or mystical bases for understanding that are more authoritative than merely human claims of knowledge (Eliade, 1959; Pals, 1996). In contrast, professional social work does not make such a claim. It claims humanistic values and perspectives and scientific information as its bases. Although social workers may work from general theories of human behavior and models of practice, these are constantly subject to revision as new empirical evidence critiques them. Further, social workers tend to be more concerned with the immediacy, variety, and practicality of client experiences and situations than with claims of universal truth.

Second, traditional religious believers, at least in the Judaic, Christian, and Islamic traditions, commonly have a primary commitment to membership in one religion and upholding of one faith, even if they are open to ecumenical and interreligious dialogue and interaction. Some religious believers may feel that proselytization and maintenance or expansion of their religious membership are their duties. Religious believers may feel that their own moral codes are divinely approved and that anyone who does not conform to them is morally insufficient and spiritually endangered. In contrast, professional social work has a primary commitment to respecting the diversity of religious and nonreligious forms of spirituality and whatever spiritual standpoint the client takes. Religious proselytization in a professional social work context is contrary to our Code of Ethics. Social workers follow the dictum, 'start where the client is,' meaning that we refrain from negative judgments or a priori assumptions about clients. We try to understand their perspectives, needs, and aspirations and help them to reach their goals on their own terms, in so far as this does not violate law or people's safety.

Thirdly, helpers and healers within religious traditions are recognized by fellow believers to have permission and sanction from both human authorities within their religious organizations and communities and also from a divine or sacred source, such as God or guiding spirit entities. Social workers' sanction to serve comes from professional and governmental standards, laws, and licensure requirements.

Sometimes, people view such differences in terms of contradiction and tension. But if social work and religion are to be brought together in dual degree programs, it would be helpful to find ways in which their differences can be complementary and lead to mutually beneficial challenges. When a student juxtaposes insights from religion and social work, the contrasts can stimulate new insights. In addition, the student may find deep commonalities between them, perhaps in part because of the religious roots of professional social work and also the common heart of compassion shared by religions and social work (Canda & Furman, 1999).

I had to sort through these contrasts and commonalities in a very personal way when I was a lay Catholic chaplain as a clinical pastoral education hospital intern in 1984, while I was engaged in doctoral social work study. I wanted to see what pastoral counseling as a field offered to enrich the social work perspective. In this situation, I was a person trained as a social worker who entered a pastoral care role. Within the hospital setting, I had the role of chaplain. This label cued patients who wished to discuss their health or personal crises in relation to their spirituality that I was willing and available to do so. Many times, within just a few minutes, patients opened up about deep feelings, religious beliefs, and reflections about God. If I had come into the patient's room with a social worker label, more likely they would have been prompted to talk about practicalities of discharge planning, or emotional and relational issues without an explicit religious or spiritual tone. For interested Catholic patients, I could also bring the sacrament of the Eucharist to share with them in prayer. This resulted in moments of spiritual intimacy quite different from anything I had experienced as a social worker.

On the other hand, the chaplain role label inhibited some patients who assumed I came to proselytize or judge them. Also, the hospital rules for job roles did not allow me to follow through with patients on psychosocial issues that were defined as belonging to social work turf. The institutional dichotomy between chaplain and social worker required me to create an artificial division within myself. I also had to regard the patient like a pie cut into slices, the hospital regulations portioning out the chaplain piece to myself and the social work piece to social workers. Eventually, I was able to learn how to work within these role distinctions. Yet, the internal and institutional dichotomization led to a sense of role tension and alienation for me and a lack of holistic relating with patients.

Similar to my experience, it is likely that students who engage in shifting between the two sides of religion and social work dual degree programs may feel times of disjoint, fragmentation, and marginalization. Students need help to connect across these two realms, within themselves, and within educational and social service programs.

It is important to note that underneath the apparent differences between clinical pastoral education and social work, there was a deep commonality. Both fields demonstrated a commitment to compassionate, knowledgeable, and skillful service that respected patients' own spiritual views. Yet in my internship, these differences were not made complementary, the commonalities were not explicitly addressed, and an integrated teamwork approach was not utilized.

My experiences lead to suggestions about ways that studies of religion and social work can provide stimulating and constructive challenges to each other when connected in dual degree programs.

How Religion Can Challenge Social Work

Both social workers and religious helpers may view their work as a form of calling in the sense of a vocation related to a deep life commitment. For religious helpers, this sense of calling may be very literal: that God or other sacred powers have called them to a life of service. Religion can remind social workers to keep their sense of calling clear, whether or not this is understood in religious terms. There is the strong example of St. Paul who found his calling when God knocked him off his high horse of egoism and violence and blinded him with a flash of light so that he could gain new sight as a person reborn in dedication to Christ (Acts 9:1-31). Social workers can keep a vivid sense of why they are on the path of service and what are the deepest motivations and purposes for their work.

Religions often have ways to symbolize the personal balance and centering in a heart of compassion and love that are necessary for transformative service. For example, Christian rose windows, Hindu and Buddhist mandalas, and First Nations' medicine wheels symbolize how we need to integrate and balance all aspects of ourselves, centered in a sacred point that connects all our aspects and all the aspects of the world (Coggins, 1990; Cunningham, 2003; Jung 1959). As social workers, we often draw on theories for practice that address the biological, psychological, social (and more recently) spiritual aspects of people. We seek holistic understandings of personal and social systems. Religious teachings can remind us to regard ourselves, our clients, and the world as wholes, to work from our own sacred centers, to live in balance personally and professionally, and to help others to do the same.

Many religions teach that genuine service involves recognizing the divine within everyone, especially the poor and oppressed. For example, the Jewish existentialist theologian, Martin Buber, described genuine relationship of love between two people as I and Thou, subject to subject, full person to full person (Canda & Furman, 1999). For Buber and many religious people, this human to human relationship is a reflection of the unconditional love of God for humanity. This insight can remind social workers not to reduce clients to diagnostic labels, symptom lists, problem categories, eligibility tests, or group stereotypes. We can be alert to the sacredness and potential for transformation within everyone and reflect this in our helping relationships.

Some religious traditions, such as Vedantic karma yoga, elaborate the nature of helping as a spiritual discipline that not only aids the ostensible recipient, but also helps the helper to increase in spiritual awareness and growth (Patel, 1987). In this sense, compassionate helping itself is intrinsically valuable, regardless of extrinsic rewards or measurable success. In the context of today's emphasis on cost effectiveness and measurable treatment outcomes, this insight can remind us not to be egoistically attached to the superficial fruits of our helping actions. We plant seeds, but we have neither the power nor the wisdom to determine ultimate outcomes. Even an apparent failure in helping could be an important turning point in someone's growth, unbeknownst to us.

Finally, religious traditions throughout the world have developed a tremendous array of helping and healing strategies, techniques, and support systems, such as meditation, prayer, ritual, symbolism, dream reflection, examination of conscience, use of sacred herbs, practices of spiritual mentoring and guidance, and customs of mutual support in religious communities (Canda & Furman, 1999; Van Hook, Hugen, & Aguilar, 2002). Social workers can learn about these, cooperate with religiously based helpers and social support systems relevant to clients, and sometimes apply them directly according to clients' wishes and with respect to the religious traditions themselves.

How Social Work Can Challenge Religion

Social work as a profession is committed to help all people achieve their full potential in the context of a just society and world. One of the concerns of social workers about religiously based service is that sometimes religious providers attach strings to their help. For example, help sometimes becomes linked with proselytization, moralistic and condescending judgments, and requirements for religious participation. Social work can challenge religion to truly accept all people where they are, to provide help without expectation of conformity, and to help all people in ways that respect all forms of diversity, including culture, religion, disability, sexual orientation, gender, and others.

Social workers, including those with a strong spiritual orientation, often work in settings that are funded by public money or that involve clients of many different religious and nonreligious forms of spirituality. Therefore, in some settings it is not appropriate to discuss religion overtly, or to display one's own religious commitment, or to offer explicit religious advice or ideas to clients. Yet spiritually sensitive social workers can regard the helping relationship and process as themselves a mode of prayer or meditation (Canda, 1990). This can remind religious persons that even without explicit religious words and actions, the way we conduct ourselves moment to moment is already prayer when done with alertness, compassion, and skillful attention to clients' own needs, strengths, and goals.

Social work blends artistry and humane values with scientific evidence and technical skill. Because we are accountable for our professional actions and the resources expended for helping, we must consider what is really helpful. This can remind religions to reflect critically on traditional ideas and practices about the causes and solutions for human problems, such as mental illness, substance abuse, and poverty. If religiously based ideas about helping do not hold up to careful scrutiny, then they need to be revised.

IMPLICATIONS FOR DESIGN OF DUAL DEGREE MASTER'S PROGRAMS

Dual degree programs should be structured to facilitate students' efforts to bring studies of religion and social work into creative integration. Allowing students to enroll in two different programs is necessary but insufficient for true integration to occur. Students need explicit organizational support and mentoring by faculty members to encourage integration of insights between the two degree programs.

First of all, students should be expected to fulfill the high educational standards of each degree program. The quality of programs should not be diluted. Each degree program will convey its own body of knowledge, intellectual tradition, values, and insights for service. Students should receive the full benefit of what the programs have to offer. However, students should not be overwhelmed by doubled bureaucratic rules, regulations, and expectations. Each program needs to create policies and procedures to facilitate administration and expedited completion of both degrees. For example, this might include formal university dual degree program formation, as in social work and religious studies within a university, or as in combined programs across a cooperating seminary and a university-based social work program. This could also include cross listing of required courses and electives relevant to both degrees that can count toward requirements in both programs. Administrative procedures for application, acceptance, and matriculation of both programs need to be coordinated and streamlined.

Faculty in each program should cross-train and collaborate. For example, faculty can take sabbaticals or exchange professorships across the two programs for their own continuing education and to familiarize themselves with the perspectives and practical workings of the programs. Faculty can develop cooperative research and community service projects, so that the strengths of both fields are combined in their work. Faculty who develop this kind of experience (or themselves have dual degrees in religion and social work) will be well prepared to administer, teach, and advise in the dual degree programs.

Faculty instructors and advisors in each program within a dual degree program should be informed about the students' participation so that they can be attentive to ways the students can connect learning across the two programs within particular courses. Students can be encouraged to do course assignments in both programs that make an explicit link between them. For example, in a religious studies course on theories of religious experience, a student could write a paper on assessment of spiritual crises in mental health settings, drawing on insights from transpersonal theory and mystical theology. In a social work practicum course (i.e., supervised service learning experience in agency settings), students could work in agencies that encourage ways to address religion and spirituality as relevant to clients, such as in religiously sponsored human service agencies, services for immigrants and refugees, hospice programs, grief and loss counseling programs, and 12-step oriented substance abuse treatment programs.

The two degree programs should require a cross-over course or other educational experience that explicitly integrates religion and social work. At a minimum, this could be a specially designed individual or group study course, tailored to the dual degree students and supervised by a faculty person (or co-taught from an instructor from each program). If there are a sufficient number of students enrolled in the dual degree program on a regular basis, a cross-over integration course could be designed as a standard offering. If this is not possible, then a course designed for the general student, but with content especially relevant to religion and social work, can include a tailored assignment for the dual degree student. For example, within social work MSW programs, a course on spirituality and social work would offer an excellent opportunity for this. If a comprehensive exam or thesis is required in either or both programs, the dual degree student should be expected to work on a topic that explicitly links concerns of the two programs.

Informal aspects of support and learning are just as crucial for a good educational experience as are formal aspects of program design. Therefore, students in dual degree programs should have academic advisors who are familiar with both programs, have a special interest in cross-disciplinary integration, and are enthusiastic to mentor dual degree students. In addition, students who participate in a dual degree program should be connected with each other socially, so that they can offer each other mutual support, encouragement, and tips for success through the program.

Mutual support can extend beyond the two directly involved programs. Faculty and students in dual degree programs around the country can form a network of mutual support and also become involved in organizations, such as the Society for Spirituality and Social Work (http://sehd.binghamton.edu/affprograms/sssw/) or the American Academy of Religion (http://www.aarweb.org/default.asp), for cross-fertilization of ideas.

CONCLUSION

The challenge of integrating perspectives of religion and social work within a dual degree program may be similar to the challenge of achieving biculturality. A First Nations elder provided a helpful metaphor for this challenge (anonymous personal communication, 1981) when he described the difficulty of living in two worlds, his Indigenous culture and the predominantly European American culture. He said that he sometimes felt like a person trying to ride downriver by standing with each foot in a different canoe. That is a situation of precarious balance and stress, unlikely to protect one from drowning. Although his cross-cultural experience is likely to have been more difficult and dramatic than that of most dual degree students, dual degree students also face the difficulty of finding balance and connection between two worlds. This is not trivial. The difficulty of connecting across religion and social work programs intellectually, emotionally, socially, and spiritually can be significant. Since students are only likely to do this because of a serious and deep interest, the effort to make the connection is likely to have profound meaning for their lives.

To continue this metaphor, dual degree programs need to offer students a catamaran. A catamaran is a sailboat with a float on either side connected to a place to sit in between. The two floats represent the two programs that lift up the student on her or his educational journey. Dual degree programs need to be designed so that the student can occupy a place between studies of religion and social work and can connect across them. Then the wind of spirit can fill the student's sail.

NOTE

The author thanks the members of his dissertation committee. Their encouragement was crucial to his career in social work: Dr. Virginia Richardson (chairperson), Dr. William Eldridge, and Dr. Daniel B. Lee.

REFERENCES

Bullis, R. K. (1996). *Spirituality in social work practice*. Washington, DC: Taylor & Francis.

Canda, E. R. (1988a). Conceptualizing spirituality for social work: Insights from diverse perspectives. *Social Thought*, *14*(1), 30-46.

Canda, E. R. (1988b). Spirituality, religious diversity, and social work practice. *Social Casework*, *69*(4), 238-247.

Canda, E. R. (1990). An holistic approach to prayer for social work practice. *Social Thought*, *16*(3), 3-13.

Canda, E. R., & Furman, L. D. (1999). *Spiritual diversity in social work practice: The heart of helping*. New York, NY: The Free Press.

Canda, E. R., Nakashima, M., Burgess, V., Russel, R., & Barfield, S. (2003). *Spiritual diversity and social work: A comprehensive bibliography with annotations, second edition.* Alexandria, VA: Council on Social Work Education Press.

Capps, W. H. (1995). *Religious studies: The making of a discipline.* Minneapolis, MN: Fortress Press.

Cnaan, R. A., Wineburg, R. J., & Boddie, S. C. (1999). *The newer deal: Social work and religion in partnership.* NY: Columbia University Press.

Coggins, K. (1990). *Alternative pathways to healing: The recovery medicine wheel.* Deerfield Beach, FL: Health Communications.

Cunningham, B. (2003). *Mandala: Journey to the center.* NY: DK Publishing.

Eliade, M. (1959). *The sacred and the profane: The nature of religion.* NY: Harper & Row.

Ellor, J. W., Netting, F. E., & Thibault, J. M. (1999). *Religious and spiritual aspects of human service practice.* Charleston, SC: University of South Carolina.

Jung, C. G. (1959). Concerning mandala symbolism. In H. Read, M. Fordham, & G. Adler (Eds.), *The collected works of C. G. Jung (vol. 9, pt. 1)* (pp. 355-390). NY: Free Press.

Pals, D. L. (1996). *Seven theories of religion.* NY: Oxford University Press.

Patel, I. (1987). *Vivekenanda's approach to social work.* Mylapore, India: Sri Ramakrishna Math.

Russel, R. (1998). Spirituality and religion in graduate social work education. In Edward R. Canda (Ed.), *Spirituality in social work: New directions.* Binghamton, NY: The Haworth Press, Inc., pp. 15-29.

Simpkinson, C., Wengell, D., & Casavant, M.J. (Eds.), (1994). *The common boundary graduate education guide: Holistic programs and resources integrating spirituality and psychology.* Bethesda, MD: Common Boundary, Inc.

Siporin, M. (1985). Current social work perspectives on clinical practice. *Clinical Social Work Journal 13*(3), 198-217.

Siporin, M. (1986). Contribution of religious values to social work and the law. *Social Thought, 12*(4), 35-50.

Van Hook, M. P., Hugen, B., & Aguilar, M. (Eds.), (2002). *Spirituality within religious traditions in social work practice.* New York, NY: Wadsworth.

Teaching About Organized Religion in Social Work: Lessons and Challenges

Ram A. Cnaan
Stephanie C. Boddie
Rivka A. Danzig

SUMMARY. It is commonly taught in schools of social work that the origin of the profession is in the humanistic principles of the many world faith traditions. However, social work education, research, and practice had disassociated themselves from religion and its contribution to the profession from as early as the days of the Charity Organization Societies (COS) in the late nineteenth century to the Social Security Act of 1935. Society, however, especially in the last two decades is marching toward greater integration between social services and organized religion. Furthermore, a large number of social workers, regardless of their personal religious affiliations, were trained to think that their religion has no relevance for their everyday professional practice. This rift, ex-

Ram A. Cnaan, PhD, and Rivka A. Danzig, PhD, are affiliated with the School of Social Work, University of Pennsylvania. Stephanie C. Boddie, PhD, is affiliated with the George Warren Brown School of Social Work, Washington University.

Address correspondence to: Ram A. Cnaan, School of Social Work, University of Pennsylvania, 3701 Locust Walk, Philadelphia, PA 19104 (E-mail: cnaan@ssw.upenn.edu).

[Haworth co-indexing entry note]: "Teaching About Organized Religion in Social Work: Lessons and Challenges." Cnaan, Ram A., Boddie, Stephanie C., and Danzig, Rivka A. Co-published simultaneously in *Journal of Religion & Spirituality in Social Work: Social Thought* (The Haworth Social Work Practice Press, an imprint of The Haworth Press, Inc.) Vol. 24, No. 1/2, 2005, pp. 93-110; and: *Social Work and Divinity* (ed: Daniel Lee, and Robert O'Gorman) The Haworth Social Work Practice Press, an imprint of The Haworth Press, Inc., 2005, pp. 93-110. Single or multiple copies of this article are available for a fee from The Haworth Document Delivery Service [1-800-HAWORTH, 9:00 a.m. - 5:00 p.m. (EST). E-mail address: docdelivery@haworthpress.com].

http://www.haworthpress.com/web/JRSSW

Digital Object Identifier: 10.1300/J377v24n01_09

tenuated in the past fifty years, has been challenged by devolutionary trends of government funding and social service delivery that encourage faith-based social service provision. It also challenged the dogmatic exclusion of religious contents in social work education. In this article, we review the place of organized religion in social work education and present our innovative course to re-link organized religion into social work curriculum.

KEYWORDS. Religion, charity organization society, social work education, faith, social service delivery

BACKGROUND

It is commonly accepted that the origins of social work are within the religious traditions and practices of the world. However, since the end of the nineteenth century the two slowly parted ways. The scant attention given by social work educators and researchers to any religion-related topic is, by now, well documented (Cnaan, Boddie, & Wineburg, 1999; Loewenberg, 1988; Magnuson, 1977). Martin Marty (1980), in a special essay in *Social Service Review*, observed that: " . . . most of the time the literature of the profession [social work] genially and serenely ignores religion" (p. 465). This rift, its aftermath, and how to overcome it are the focus of this paper.

It is our view that there is a need for social work professionals who integrate both religious understanding and social work skills and values. We believe that schools of social work should take a leading role in educating the next cadre of providers of social services and produce graduates that are informed about how to work with and within faith-based social service agencies as well as to help people who are serious about their religion. We should also make religious people welcome in our schools and make their belief systems accepted and respected.

In this paper we will first demonstrate that the rift between social work and religion really exists. We report findings from various sources showing that the magnitude of coverage of religion in social work literature is negligible. We then proceed to detail how social work educators and researchers first called for total disregarding of religion, especially in the middle of the twentieth century, the era post passage of the Social Security Act. An important question that often arises is why should social work pay tribute to organized religion and religious beliefs. The third major section of this article deals with this dilemma and provides convincing support to the need to reattach the two camps. Finally, we provide information about our attempt to bridge this rift. We developed a course designed to educate interested students about the importance and dilemmas involved in working for or working in tandem with religious organizations and religious people. We hope that this modest beginning will be of interest for others and a model for replication or improvement.

Actual Coverage of Religion in Social Work Literature

To examine the extent to which social work education has addressed organized religion and faith-based social services, Cnaan, Boddie, and Wineburg (1999) used five different approaches.

(1) *Abstracts of Papers Presented at the Annual Meeting of the Council on Social Work Education:* These authors analyzed abstracts of all papers presented at five Annual Program Meetings (APM) of the Council on Social Work Education (CSWE) (1990-1994) for content on religion. Of the 1,500 papers presented at the APM, only 30 papers (2%) dealt with religion and service delivery. Most of these had to do with the history of service provision, while others described ways in which a spiritual focus might help in the therapeutic settings. Sectarian-based or denominational services received little attention. Only two papers dealt with the contemporary concerns of religious-based social services. Similar results were obtained by these authors when studying 1997 and 1998 APMs.

(2) *Articles Abstracted in the Social Work Abstracts:* The Social Work Abstracts database, designed specifically for social workers, lists more than 35,000 sources for the period of 1977 to March 1997. In this database, these authors identified 220 sources (.0063%), mostly articles, that contained the term "religion" and "social work." In many of these articles, however, the term religion referred to spirituality and not to organized religion or religious-based social service. When they excluded: (a) articles/dissertations/publications that did not address religion; (b) articles published in a journal from another discipline such as sociology, psychology, criminology, or from religious journals such as *Social Thought* or *Journal for the Scientific Study of Religion*; and (c) those published outside the United States, the number of pertinent sources decreased to thirty-eight

(.001%). These findings, echoed Joseph (1987) who noted that "The social work literature barely touches these areas [spirituality] and does not present in a systematic fashion personal development in relation to belief in God" (p. 16). Furthermore, Joseph noted that "the major social work journals contained only a few articles on religion, which may reflect an ambivalence around religion or its isolation in practice to religious settings."

(3) *Textbooks Used in Social Work Education:* A review of the 20 most commonly used textbooks in courses of social policy and social welfare history and philosophy revealed that, with few exceptions, the texts made no mention of any congregational or sectarian aspect of social work with the exception of the obligatory nod to Charity Organization Societies (COSs). Any textual references to religious-based social services ended with the Great Depression and the Social Security Act of 1935. The main emphasis in the texts, however, was on issues of state and federal legislation. More recently, *Dimensions of Social Welfare Policy*, by Gilbert and Terrell (2002), and *American Social Welfare Policy: A Pluralistic Approach,* by Karger and Stoesz (2002), specifically highlight organized religion as a vital social institution.

(4) *Course Outlines Used in Schools of Social Work:* Cnaan, Boddie, and Wineburg (1999) further analyzed 50 social welfare course outlines posted at the 1993 and 1994 APM meetings. Only five course outlines (10%) mentioned religiously-affiliated social service provisions, and again it was in the context of either the history of the profession or the threats to social work from the extreme religious right. A notable exception was religiously-affiliated schools of social work which offer courses in issues such as church social work.

(5) *Review of the National Association of Social Work Yearbooks and Encyclopedias of Social Work:* Finally, these authors reviewed the cover given to religious social service in the *Social Work Year Books* and *Encyclopedias of Social Work*. In most of the issues of the *Encyclopedia of Social Work*, the origins of social work were attributed to the settlement movement or the Charity Organization Society and not to religious origins. Instead, social work provided by religious-based organizations was delineated according to religious groups: Catholic, Jewish, Mormon, and Protestant. Each group is presented with unique values, understanding of the nature of man, and reason for helping. In later editions of the *Encyclopedia of Social Work*, religious organization are classified as one group. From the 1965-1968 edition onward, social services provided by religious-based organizations are referred to as religious sponsorship. In the 1971,1977, and 1987 editions, religious-based social services are categorized as sectarian

agencies. In 1997, with more activity and interest in social work by religious organizations, the nineteenth edition and supplement gives more attention to the work of religious organizations: Church Social Work, Christian Social Work, Jewish Communal Services, and Spirituality.

These findings are not new. In 1980 Martin Marty (1980) noted that: "Schools of social work rarely include curricular references to the religious roots or implications of the profession or to the manifestly religious contexts of most of the beneficiaries of social welfare activities" (p. 465). These findings suggest that for a long time is was uncommon to allow religious contexts in social work curriculum. In fact, many religious people felt uncomfortable with social work's over-emphasis of liberal-humanistic values and had to hide their true religious sentiments and perspectives (Streets, 1997). Similar expression of compassion for people in need were accepted secularly but frowned upon if used as part of a biblical or religious text.

Social Work Changing View of Organized Religion

In 1962, Herbert Bisno proposed a secularly oriented social work practice. He based this on key principles in social work, such as self-determination and client-oriented intervention, which emphasize flexible service according to each client's needs. Bisno asserted that religious perspectives contradict such principles and hence suggested the neglect of religion in social work circles:

> The church . . . has continued to hold firmly to the existence of certain fixed unchanging moral principles, and this, in the nature of things, she must continue to do. The possession of these principles must have a far-reaching effect on the endeavors of Catholic social workers; for in the Catholic scheme of things such principles not only determine the pattern of our individual lives; they determine to a large extent our relationships with others, the social program at which we aim and the objectives we endeavor to place before those in whose behalf we work. (p. 92)

We are not sure if Bisno had predicted the scandal involving pedophile priests, but he assessed that religion is so rigid that social work will be unable to cooperate with it. Bisno further noted that Catholic and other religious social workers must oppose on moral grounds clients' requests for abortion, contraception, divorce, or gay and lesbian relationships. Bisno therefore called for a separation of the new profession from its religious roots.

In 1952, the same year in which *Philosophy of Social Work* was published, the American Association of Schools of Social Work (now the CSWE) adopted its first Curriculum Policy Statement. This curriculum statement made no reference to spirituality or religion, as its drafters assumed that the humanistic emphasis of social work spanned all human needs and required areas of knowledge (Spencer, 1957; 1961). Spencer asserted that most social work educators were weary of any presentation of religion in social work curriculum as being unnecessary and illogical.

In recent years more calls were made for the inclusion of content on organized religion in social work education. Since the 1980s Robert Wineburg (1990-91; 1993; 1994; 1996) began studying faith-based organizations in Greensboro, N.C. He found that the three largest networks of religious social services–Catholic Charities, Jewish Family and Children Services, and the Salvation Army–not only expanded during this period but also began to hire BSWs and MSWs as a matter of course. In 1990, Netting, Thibault, and Ellor called for the inclusion of organized religion in social work education on the basis that organized religion is an important force in community change, in working with social and health services, and in policy development and implementation. They pointed out that: "Even when the unit of analysis is a church-related social service agency, it is helpful for the social worker to understand the agency's theological foundations, its formal structure relationship to the parent religious body, and its potential for either attracting clients or frightening them away" (p. 15). Consequently, they proposed that macro practice courses, those dealing with planning, administration, policy and so forth, include content about organized religion.

Allen-Meares (1989) studied adolescent sexuality and teenage parents among the African-American community. Allen-Meares proposed that church youth programs should teach youth "responsible decision-making and interpersonal skills by using realistic role playing and situations that they will encounter in life" (p. 141). She used three arguments to justify her position on recruiting churches to solve a social work problem. One is that more than half of America's black community have strong ties to the church. Another is that pastors are also community and educational leaders. Finally, the church is the social institution where both parents and children participate.

Two recent books, one by Cnaan, Boddie, and Wineburg (1999), and one by Canda and Furman (1999), reflect the newly emerged role of religion in social work. They discuss spirituality in a balanced manner and suggest numerous ways by which social workers can use spirituality in practice. Cnaan and his colleagues called for a cautious and limited partnership between social work and religion. They also suggested that many social workers and their clients are religious. Many came to social work for religious motives and many clients gain strength and mutual support through their religious beliefs (see also Sheridan & Amato von Hemert, 1999).

The long-standing debate over religious content in social work education was highlighted in 1994 when *Journal of Social Work Education* published two articles debating the question: "Should social work education address religion issues?" Katherine Amato von Hemert suggested that ignoring the issue of religion causes social work practitioners to forget their "whole self" and act in a stilted manner. Her position was that not only should social work collaborate with religious-based organizations, but also that the religious values and beliefs of social workers and their clients should be incorporated into practice and into the training of future social workers. James Clark argued that neglect of religious issues is not an ethical compromise, and that religious issues should be raised by the profession only when they are relevant. He further asserted that "Social work must resist reactionary efforts to redefine complex social problems as the result of moral and spiritual failure, of specific individuals or the nation as a whole" (p. 11). Clark's position suggests much more than is actually stated. While he contends–and we agree–that victims of society should not be defined as moral failures, he also defines working with religious-based social services as archaic and reactionary. In this latter respect, Clark represents the views of those social workers who see only one side of the religious community–that of the Moral Majority and the extreme conservatives–and not the many who want to better the world.

What is most astonishing is that most social workers are quite sympathetic to religious issues. In a survey of practitioners conducted by M. Vincentia Joseph (1988), most respondents (more than 80%) reported that they believed it was important to focus attention on religion in social work practice, yet more than 50 percent said they rarely or never dealt with religious issues in their practice. While many students are placed in field-placement in faith-based agencies, they are rarely provided with training relevant for practice in these agencies. Were they child-welfare or old-home agencies, the students were obliged to study child-welfare or gerontology as the case may be. Religious agencies are frequently used as field placement sites ranging from Catholic Charities to small Baptist homeless shelters, from Lutheran homes to synagogues, and from Salvation Army centers to faith-based local coalitions. In all cases the students are expected to bridge the social work milieu, which is largely anti-clerical, with the religious nature of the field placement on their own.

The Rationale for the Inclusion of Religious Content in Social Work Education

When one proposes to change the way curriculum is designed a good rationale should be articulated. It is our contention that social work should embrace religious issues and make them part of the required curriculum. Maybe the key reason to incorporate issues of religion was stated by Marty (1997): "religion motivates most killing in the world today" but also "contributes to most healing in the world today" (p. 20). Indeed this immense power to motivate so many people so powerfully should not be ignored by any social science discipline.

Social work and its practitioners will most likely be affected by the changing political and legal climate. With the passage of Section 104 of welfare reform (a.k.a., charitable choice), many more services will be provided under religious auspices (Cnaan & Boddie, 2002; Sherman, 2000). The political climate of the past twenty years calls for moral judgment and moral and religious-based social interventions. More and more public services are contracted out to religious providers and it is now legal to provide social and educational service via religious providers while they maintain their religious message. In January, 2001 President Bush made faith-based help for the poor his key domestic policy. By establishing the White House Office of Faith Based and Community Initiatives (OFBCI) the president demonstrated that care for the neediest members of our society will be expected to come from the local faith-based organizations, and mainly from congregations. Clearly, social workers need to be educated and informed regarding these new trends and policies as well as prepared to work in these auspices.

Furthermore, the United States is a very religious country where religion is important to people and where communities of interests are drawn along congregational boundaries. The United States is the most religious country among all modern democracies. For example, the World Value Survey conducted from 1990 to 1993 found that more people in the United States (82%) defined themselves as religious than do those in any other county (*The Economist*, 1995). In a 1993 CNN/USA Today/Gallup poll, 71 percent of Americans reported membership in a church or synagogue, and 41 percent reported attendance at a church or synagogue in the seven days prior to the poll (McAneny & Saad, 1993). Recently, the latest Gallup Index of Leading Religious Indicators, based on a series of surveys conducted in 2000, reveals that Americans are more religious today than ten years ago, but less than in the 1950s. Over 90 percent of those interviewed believe in God and state a clear religious preference. More than two-thirds (68.2%) belong to an organized place of worship and over half (58.7%) report that their religion is important in their lives. Finally, two thirds (64.9%) report that religion offers answers to life problems (Gallup, 2001). In a recent study, Cnaan, Gelles, and Sinha (2002), based on a national representative sample of 2,004 teens, found that among young Americans religion is as strong as among adults. An overwhelming majority (83.7%) reported that religion is important in their lives. Two-thirds (66.8%) reported attending a place of worship for prayer purposes in the month prior to the interview. And two-fifths (41.2%) reported to be members of a youth social group that is part of a congregation or a religious organization.

Not only are Americans religious, they also trust their religious leaders. Kilpatrick and Holland (1990) noted that "Ministers are more often sought out for guidance in resolving personal problems than are social workers" (p. 129). Allen-Meaeas, as discussed above, suggested including clergy in campaigns for working to minimize teen pregnancy as the clergy are accepted community leaders. Cnaan, Boddie, and Wineburg (1999) noted many instances where local clergy serve as community leaders/representatives and work to solve key community problems. Gelles and Straus (1989) found that battered women reported that they often consulted clergy. Even the latest cases of sexual abuse by Catholic priests throughout the country is indicative of the basic trust people have toward the clergy. The fact that some priests could have continued to molest children while the families could not have believed can happen only amidst a foundation of deep trust. Clergy, albeit human beings and as such capable of misusing trust, are perceived and expected to be exemplary in their behavior and morality.

Furthermore, clergy and active congregational members are the closest to people in the community and are familiar with members' expectations and needs. When we talk about using reliable informants in community practice and conducting needs assessment at the community level, there is no better source than the various religious institutions. They are the most common organizations in any neighborhood and often are the most familiar with the real needs of neighbors as they keep in touch with many local families.

In America the strongest and most vibrant communities are the local religious congregations (Cnaan et al., 2002). In these communities social capital is gained and meaningful interactions are taking place. Almost half of the population meets weekly or more often and share face to face interactions. Members of congregations are familiar with each other, plan activities together, engage in mutual fellowship, and often serve people in need. Cnaan and Boddie (2001) reported that in Philadelphia, nine out of ten congregations, regardless of income or religion, provide at least one social service to better the life of people in the community. And these services are often aimed at people who are not members of the congregation.

As noted above, many social workers practice under religious auspices or in collaboration with religious-based social services. Many other social workers are affiliated with religious groups and/or use spiritually oriented methods in their practice (Sheridan & Amato-von Hemert, 1999; Loewenberg, 1988). Social work students are often placed in faith-based organizations. In fact, in one school, Cnaan, Boddie, and Wineburg (1999) report that one of every eight student is placed in fieldwork in either first or second year in a religious-based social service organization. The range of such agencies extends from large agencies such as Jewish Family and Children Services, Catholic Social Services, and Lutheran Child Services to small local religious congregations in West Philadelphia. Yet, we have very little knowledge and understanding of the unique nature of these agencies and students are not prepared to practice in these agencies.

For a large number of people, religious beliefs and practices are the source of strength and survival. People who face serious hardships such as major illnesses, job loss, traumas, or extreme poverty often find strength and hope in their religious beliefs. Clinging to God and finding solace in fulfilling God's wish helps them cope with the situation and master the coping mechanism needed. Ignoring the power of belief is an erroneous social work practice and students should be taught how to unleash beliefs where appropriate.

Teaching about organized religion and how to practice in this environment is in line with the Code of Ethics issued by the National Association of Social Workers, which states clearly in section 4.02 (discrimination) that:

> Social workers should not practice, condone, or collaborate with any form of discrimination on the basis of race, ethnicity, national

origin, color, sex, sexual orientation, age, marital status, political belief, religion, or mental or physical disability. (pp. 22-23)

Finally, religion can be a source of opposition to social work values and policies. While religion can be a liberating and pro-social force, as in the case of the Civil Rights movement, it can also be in inhibiting force. Campaigns against rights and protection to gay and lesbians often come from religious circles and are often anchored in religious theology. Similarly, attempts to limit women control over their clothes, body, freedom, and reproduction are generated from extreme religious circles. International and national acts of terrorism are often explained and glorified by religious differences and fanaticism. Conflicts in the Middle East or North Ireland and the tragedy of September 11 are all taking their roots and solace in religious differences that explain human differences and justify hatred and violence. Organized religion is not a pure matter and it contains many types and variations–some most humane and caring and some most extremist and hateful. But, ignoring either is unwise.

This sparse scholarship on religion in social work deprives social work educators, scholars, and practitioners alike of the opportunity to consider important facts and trends that are critical to the present and future of the profession. This has a bearing on effective service delivery in the long term. We therefore argue that social work must pay more attention to its own roots which are firmly grounded in religious traditions, as the following section will show. While the care for those in need is addressed by both social work and religious organizations, few social work programs integrate social work, religion, and spirituality. Most schools fail to address the nexus between social work education and practice under religious auspices.

Training Students to Work in and with Faith-Based Social Services

Organized religion and faith will play a major role in the tapestry of publicly funded social services and in the quality of life of individuals nationwide. How, then, can we train new cohorts of social workers into being competent in addressing people's religious needs as well as working with faith-based providers to alleviate human misery? We need to enable future social workers to be able to work with religious leaders from a variety of faith traditions and to be able to manage and practice in such agencies.

The means to achieve these goals are many and diverse. They range from a one time lecture on the topic in an introductory class (policy, practice, or HBSE) to a full fledged five year dual degree jointly offered by seminaries and schools of social work. Our approach was to develop and teach a comprehensive course "Practicing and Managing Social Work in Religious Contexts."[1] The advantage of this approach is that a group of social work students receive an in-depth familiarity with the topic. The disadvantage is that only a self-select few receive this content knowledge. It should be noted that the school attitude towards this course proceeded from originally disapproving the course as a regular part of the curriculum (first year it was taught as an experimental course) to its full adoption and for inclusion of religious contents in introduction to policy, practice, and HSBE courses. In fact, in the past two years all first year students receive a class-wide lecture in introduction to social policy that covers faith-based social service delivery and charitable choice and informs students of the place of organized religion in the complex network of social service delivery systems.

This focus of this course centers on three key issues that are relevant for social work and religion: (1) social work as a profession advocating the inclusion and understanding of all aspects of human diversity and integrate them in education, practice, and research; (2) social work students learning by use of "the whole self" which includes spirituality and religious beliefs of practitioners and clients alike (Danzig, 1986; 1995); and (3) recognizing the need for social work administration and planning for religious-based social services organizations (Cnaan, Boddie, & Wineburg, 1999). Indeed, the class sessions and class discussions revolve around these three pillars and serve the practice need of both micro and macro practice students. When the class discusses a client's request to pray with the practitioner we discuss relevant social work values and rules as well as agency policies. We also assess what it means to the client and to the practitioner and how to negotiate with clients the meaning of prayers in clinical settings. Similarly, when we discuss policies related to services provision we discuss the human spirituality and religious clients' preferences and how they are affected by the policies or how non-religious clients may react to religious symbols and practices incorporated by faith-based providers.

For students who practice or may practice in a faith-based social service agency, special attention was given to the dilemma of what is of a greater precedent: Agency authority or religious authority (Chaves, 1993; Jeavons & Cnaan, 1997). Students are introduced to the tension existing in agencies that have to meet budgetary obligations while at the same time abide by theological and religious doctrines. Similarly, we worked with students to process and explore issues of personal, religious, and professional value conflicts and their resolution. Overall, the course aimed for a balance between universalistic beliefs and particularistic faiths and practices related to religion and spirituality for social work students in their direct and macro practice field assignments (Danzig, 1995). The curriculum for this special educational program drew from existing written material such as Canda, and Furman (1999), Garland (1994) and Loewenberg's (1988) books as well as our own books and articles.

The class used a dedicated list serve on which students are required to log at least ten semestrial one-page reactions to the weekly reading or reflections from their field practice. While in the first few weeks each student posts his or her weekly log irrespective of others, the professors use these logs to enhance the class discussion. Usually, from the fourth week onward students read each other's logs and discuss comments made by others. It is quite common for the class to become engaged in a debate over a topic raised by one student and then to bring the topic to fruition through a class discussion. As of the first week it is made clear that the class will respectfully accept every view point and no one will be harassed for any opinion they post or present in class–similarly, no one can be rude or condescending. Furthermore, every religious term used has to be explained assuming that people from other faith-traditions will not be familiar with it. This practice, which is extensively emphasized by the professors in the early part of the semester, allows students to openly and comfortably enquire about religious practices with which they are unfamiliar, but curious. Jewish students explained the essence of Yom Kippur and a Muslim student explained the five pillars of Islam.

Students are asked to write a final paper on topics of their choice. The papers, which are also presented in class, are required to deal with a topic that is relevant to social work and religion. As such, new topics are brought to the attention of the class and our common knowledge is extended. The following topics are illustrative examples: The relevance of the black church to inner-city at-risk youth, religion and well-being in aging, clinical social work and the Christian social worker, Christian therapy, the Jewish component of service delivery in Jewish agencies, interfaith relations and dialogue, religion and philanthropic behavior, religion and correctional institutions, the role of black religious-based organizations in social work, organized religion versus spirituality in a hospice, societal issues with homosexuality in the church, social workers' need to address the spiritual dimension of a person living with AIDS, schizophrenic delusions and religion, faith-based partners in advocating against the death penalty, Islam and service to humanity, exploring church-social services partnerships, student involvement in community outreach of an African-American church, religion and abortion, ethics in Jewish services, church, gender, and social work, the spiritual perspective in social work, the impact and place of religion in social work, charitable choice and congregation-based ministries, implementing Taoism in addressing the affects of stigmatization in the therapeutic process in religious agencies, organizational issues in developing a congregation-based community program, faith-based community development, marketing engagement theory and Hillel's approach to engaging Jewish students, addressing gender issues in leadership in congregations, developing faith-based partners at Pennsylvania Prison Society, studying the outreach of mosques in Philadelphia, Catholic social justice: history, theology, and practice, religion in public schools, and volunteerism in American communities. These topics were selected by the students as relevant to their practice or interests and are indicative of the many ways in which social work and religion cross cut each other daily, both for clients and practitioners.

In order to make the course more relevant to the students and the school, we applied a few additional educational methods. First, we invited a group of external guest presenters to present additional world views or their research or practice to the students. This method enhanced class discussion and exposed the students to a wider range of perspectives. Among the speakers are leaders in the area of social work and religion while others are managers or scholars of faith-based social welfare. We also used the course to support the school's chapter of the Society for Spirituality and Social Work. Often a guest lecturer to the class made a separate presentation to the society. As such the subject topic became better integrated with other school activities and student groups and the impact of the course was amplified. Further, we increased the link between the class and the students' field placement by requiring students to make presentations in their field agencies as well as by asking the field instructors to evaluate the student's integration of course material and their presentations at their field practice agency. As such the course was visible and its impact way beyond the walls of the classroom.

Over a five-year period there were 46 students that successfully completed this course. These students identified themselves as agnostic, secular, Christian, Buddhist, Muslim, Catholic, and Jewish. These students were both macro and micro practice students and the course was designated as "practice elective" to both sets of students. The course evaluation by students, as relating to relevance to social practice, ranged from 4.5 to 4.9 on a scale ranging from 1 (not at all relevant) to 5 (very relevant). Furthermore, the overall satisfaction from this class ranged from 4.6 to 5.0 and the course is consistently among the highest rated courses in the school.

The feedback from the students, their field supervisors, and the practice professors indicate that the course is perceived most positively. Letters from field supervisors indicate that through our students we opened the door for open discussions on the role of religion in their agencies. This was most noticeable and appreciated post-September 11, 2001. Many agencies contacted us to discuss how to conduct public prayers that are all inclusive and how to allow open discussions about religion, fanaticism, and tolerance. The key issue was that the topic was openly discussed and social workers in their agencies were open to deal with issues of religion as they do with other topics.

CONCLUSION

In this article we wanted to establish the fact that after almost 100 years of increased disengagement of social work and religion there are sure signs of renewed realignment. These signs should not be ignored as archaic and irrelevant but be viewed as a chance for reinvigorating the field of caring for those in need. These signs represent a chance for coupled efforts in helping the poor and needy as more resources, more providers, and two perspectives, the liberal-humanistic of social work and theological of all world religions can be harnessed. In order for social work to influence the manner by which social services will be provided by faith-based providers and to better help clients for whom religion is an important part of their lives, we need to train social workers to be competent and comfortable in collaborating with religious issues.

Of the many approaches to include religion in our curriculum, we elected to develop a special course. The course is offered as an elective and after five years of teaching we feel that a solid curriculum was establish and the feedback from students, field instructors, and practice faculty is most encouraging. We would love to see more aspects of the curriculum incorporating aspects of religion and spirituality and see in this course only a small beginning. We would also wish for other schools to adopt similar courses and for the course to be tested in other parts of the country.

The course discussed in this article will continue to evolve. New students and new professors will shape it in various modes. However, in a country as religious as the United States teaching of religious issues to social workers should be the norm and not an innovative curricular achievement. As long as articles like this celebrate an elective course, religion is an implant rather than an integral part of social work. However, the road for such integration starts with a course like this and we call on others to join our journey.

NOTE

Interested readers may obtain copies of the course outline from the first author.

REFERENCES

Allen-Meares, P. (1989). Adolescent sexuality and premature parenthood: Role of the black church in prevention. *Journal of Social Work and Sexuality, 8* (1), 133-142.

Bisno, H. (1952). *The philosophy of social work.* Washington, DC: Public Affairs Press.

Canda, E. R., & Furman, L. D. (1999). *Spiritual diversity in social work practice.* New York: Free Press.

Canda, E. R., & Furman, L. D. (1999). *Spiritual diversity in social work practice: The heart of helping.* New York: Free Press.

Chaves, M. (1993). Denominations as dual structures: An organizational analysis. *Sociology of Religion, 54,* 147-169.

Clark, J., & Amato von-Hemert, K. (1994). Should social work education address religious issues? *Journal of Social Work Education, 30,* 7-17.

Cnaan, R. A., & Boddie, S. C. (2001). Philadelphia census of religious congregations' involvement in social service delivery. *Social Service Review 75,* 559-589.

Cnaan, R. A., & Boddie, S. C. (2002). Charitable Choice and faith-based welfare: A call for social work. *Social Work, 47,* 244-235.

Cnaan, R. A., with Boddie, S. C., Handy, F., Yancey, G. I., & Schneider, R. (2002). *The invisible caring hand: American congregations and the Provision of welfare.* New York: New York University Press.

Cnaan, R. A., with Boddie, S. C., & Wineburg, R. J. (1999). *The newer deal: Social work and religion in partnership.* New York: Columbia University Press.

Cnaan, R. A., Gelles, R. J., & Sinha, J. W. (2002). Youth and Religion: The Gameboy generation goes to "church." Unpublished paper. University of Pennsylvania, School of Social Work, The Program for Organized Religion and Social Work.

Council on Social Work Education. (1996). *Handbook of accreditation standards and procedures* (4th ed.). Alexandria, VA: CSWE.

Danzig, R. A. (1986). Religious values versus professional values: Dichotomy or dialectic? *The Jewish Social Work Forum, 22* (Spring), 41-53.

Danzig, R. A. (1995). The battered Jewish family. In N. Linzer et al. (Eds.), *Crisis and continuity* (39-52). New York: KTAV.

The Economist, (1995, July 8). The counter-attack of God. *The Economist*, 19-21.

Gallup, G., Jr. (2001). Americans more religious now than ten years ago, but less so than in 1950s and 1960s. Press release by the Gallup Organization, Princeton, NJ. Also: *http://www.gallup.com/poll/releases/pr010329.asp*

Garland, D. R. (1994). *Church agencies: Caring for children and families in crisis*. Washington, DC: Child Welfare League of America.

Gelles, R., & Straus, M. (1989). *Intimate violence: The causes and consequences of abuse in the American family*. New York: Touchstone.

Gilbert, N., &, Terrell, P. (2002). *Dimensions of social welfare policy* (5th ed.). Boston: Allyn and Bacon.

Jeavons, T., & Cnaan, R. A. *(1997). The formation, transitions, and evolution of small religious organizations. Nonprofit and Voluntary Sector Quarterly, 26*, s62-s84.

Joseph, M. V. (1987). The religious and spiritual aspects of clinical practice: A neglected dimension of social work. *Social Thought, 13* (1), 12-23.

Karger, H., & Stoesz, D. (2002). *American social welfare policy: A pluralist approach* (4th ed.), Boston: Allyn and Bacon.

Loewenberg, F. M. (1988). *Religion and social work practice in contemporary American society*. New York: Columbia University Press.

Magnuson, N. A. (1977). *Salvation in the slums: Evangelical social work, 1865-1920*. Metuchen, NJ: Scarecrow Press.

Marty, M. E. (1980). Social service: Godly and Godless. *Social Service Review, 54*, 463-481.

Marty, M. E. (1997, September). An exuberant adventure: The academic study and teaching of religion. *Religious Studies News*, 20, 48.

McAneny, L., & Saad, L. (1993). Strong ties between religion commitment and abortion views. *The Gallup Poll Monthly, No. 331*, 35-43.

National Association of Social Workers. (1996). *Code of ethics*. Washington, DC: NASW.

Netting, E. F., Thibault, J. M., & Ellor, J. W. (1990). Integrating the content of organized religion into macropractice courses. *Journal of Social Work Education, 26*, 15-24.

Sheridan, M. J. (1992). Practitioners' personal and professional attitudes and behaviors toward religion and spirituality: Issues for education and practice. *Journal of Social Work Education, 28*, 190-204.

Sheridan, M. J. (1994). Inclusion of content on religion and spirituality in the social work curriculum. *Journal of Social Work Education, 30*, 363-376.

Sheridan, M. J., & Amato von Hemert, K. (1999). The role of religion and spirituality in social work education and practice: A survey of student views and experiences. *Journal of Social Work Education, 35* (1), 125-141.

Sherman, A. (2000). *The growing impact of charitable choice*. Washington, DC: Center for Public Justice.

Spencer, S. W. (1957). Religious and spiritual values in social work. *Social Casework, 38*, 519-526.

Spencer, S. W. (1961). What place has religion in social work education? *Social Service Review, 35*, 161-170.

Streets, F. J. (1997). *Religious values and social work education: Conflicts and outcomes*. Unpublished doctoral dissertation. New York: Yeshiva University.

Wineburg, R. J. (1990-91). A community study on the ways religious congregations support individuals and human service network. *The Journal of Applied Social Sciences, 15* (1), 51-74.

Wineburg, R. J. (1993) Social policy, service development, and religious organizations, *Nonprofit Management & Leadership, 3*, 283-299.

Wineburg, R. J. (1994). A longitudinal case study of religious congregations in local human service delivery. *Nonprofit and Voluntary Sector Quarterly, 23*, 159-169.

Wineburg, R. J. (1996). An investigation of religious support of public and private agencies in one community in an era of retrenchment. *Journal of Community Practice, 3* (2), 35-55.

Does a Dual Degree Make a Difference in Social Work: An Empirical Study

Holly B. Nelson-Becker

SUMMARY. The purpose of this mixed method study was to examine the professional integration of religion and spirituality by two groups of MSW level graduates from a large midwestern private research university with a joint degree program. The Dual Degree group consisted of all graduates with a second master's degree in religion/divinity. The second MSW-only group was a random sample matched by gender and year of graduation with the Dual Degree group. Survey questionnaires were mailed to 124 graduates with a response rate of 65%, or 81 graduates. Forty-five respondents were Dual Degree graduates while 36 had only the MSW. Obtaining advanced university or seminary education in religion is correlated with different perspectives on social work practice. Dual Degree graduates are more likely to ask about client religious views and to have a richer context for practice in this domain. *[Article copies available for a fee from The Haworth Document Delivery Service: 1-800-HAWORTH. E-mail address: <docdelivery@haworthpress.com> Website: <http://www.HaworthPress.com> © 2005 by The Haworth Press, Inc. All rights reserved.]*

Holly B. Nelson-Becker, PhD, is Assistant Professor, University of Kansas, School of Social Welfare, 1545 Lilac Lane, Lawrence, KS 66044 (E-mail: hnelson@ku.edu).

The author wishes to thank Dr. Elsie Pinkston, University of Chicago, for advising this pre-dissertation study. The author also thanks Dr. Ed Canda for encouragement to publish this data.

[Haworth co-indexing entry note]: "Does a Dual Degree Make a Difference in Social Work: An Empirical Study." Nelson-Becker, Holly B. Co-published simultaneously in *Journal of Religion & Spirituality in Social Work: Social Thought* (The Haworth Social Work Practice Press, an imprint of The Haworth Press, Inc.) Vol. 24, No. 1/2, 2005, pp. 111-124; and: *Social Work and Divinity* (ed: Daniel Lee, and Robert O'Gorman) The Haworth Social Work Practice Press, an imprint of The Haworth Press, Inc., 2005, pp. 111-124. Single or multiple copies of this article are available for a fee from The Haworth Document Delivery Service [1-800-HAWORTH, 9:00 a.m. - 5:00 p.m. (EST). E-mail address: docdelivery@haworthpress.com].

http://www.haworthpress.com/web/JRSSW

Digital Object Identifier: 10.1300/J377v24n01_10

KEYWORDS. Dual degree religion programs, religion, spirituality, social work

Social work as a profession traces its origins to the religious and philanthropic motivation that formed the Charity Organization Society and the settlement house movement in the late nineteenth and early twentieth centuries (Marty, 1980). However, it has only recently begun to recover and explore what may be described in Jungian terms as a shadow attribute: its religious sensibility. Previously, holding religious affiliation or seeking additional religious education was viewed as a bias that kept mental health practitioners from acting in a value-free manner with clients. Social work now recognizes that in reality no practitioners are without values. It is perhaps more important to understand the foundation of the value structures that inform one's practice–to be conscious of how these may be facilitative or obstructive in building a therapeutic alliance with clients and providing help. Religion and spirituality both supply value sets that range on a continuum from fundamentalist to liberal positions and result from a combination of personal traditions, experience, and education. Does having university or seminary level religious education shape an MSW level social worker to address spiritual and religious issues more, less, or differently with clients than MSW social workers without that preparation?

In recent years, more graduate students of social work are arriving at the university with the intention of also pursuing graduate study in religion. Some have earned a theological or religious degree first, and then found themselves drawn toward social work because of its concern with social justice and marginalized people. Others experience a sense of calling, perhaps heightened by social work's historical appeal to meeting social and individual needs, that leads them later to study religion in formal way. Students choosing each of these pathways do so because they decide that each discipline has something to say to the other, but they have struggled with that integrative process. Some universities have established prescribed relationships between the departments of social work and religion, as well as nearby seminaries, that allow cross-credit for certain coursework and decrease time to graduation (e.g., reduction from five years to obtain a Master of Divinity and a MSW/AM degree to four years in a joint degree program). Clients may be defined in the traditional social work venue as individuals seeking services or in a broader context as parishioners or congregants.

LITERATURE REVIEW

Spirituality, conceptualized as a dimension that intersects religion but is also different from it, is a current topic in social work literature (Canda & Furman, 1999; Carroll, 2001; Goldberg, 1996). Spirituality is viewed in three nested concentric circles as the center of a person; one equal dimension among the psychological, biological, sociological, and spiritual aspects; or as wholeness of the person in relationship with all (Canda & Furman, 1999). From a religious studies perspective, religion is viewed as the overarching dimension of an individual; spirituality is but one aspect (D.S. Browning, personal communication, July, 1999). Religion for social work is circumscribed as an institutional pattern of beliefs, practices, and values that incorporate spirituality and is shared by a community (Canda, 1997). These different interpretations by social work and religion disciplines could lead to contradictions within graduates trained in both unless they choose to privilege one position.

Published studies have surveyed MSW students on the role of religion and spirituality in social work education and practice (Furman, 1995; Herzog & Russel, 1995; Rizer & McColley, 1996; Sheridan & Amato-von Hemert, 1999). Other studies have investigated practitioner views on religion and spirituality both inside social work (Canda, 1988; Bullis, 1996; Derezotes, 1995; Derezotes & Evans, 1995; Joseph, 1987, 1988; Sheridan & Bullis, 1991; Sheridan, Bullis, Adcock, Berlin, & Miller, 1992) and in related professions (Bergin & Jensen, 1990; Shafranske & Malony, 1990). However, no studies to date have compared MSW-only graduates with Dual Degree graduates on their integration of religion and spirituality in practice. This paper will address some of the findings from one investigation that sought to bridge this gap.

Study Questions

This study of joint or combined degree MSW graduates (those who also hold a Master of Arts in Religion or in Divinity) considered how practice with clients might vary from social work practice by a MSW-only graduate. Joint and combined degree graduates in religion are referred to in this paper as Dual Degree graduates. Questions were asked about employment setting and employment trajectory, clients served, education and training in religion and spirituality, values held regarding religion and spirituality, and personal approaches to problem-solving using religion and spirituality. In addition, questions were posed about spiritual strategies used with clients. Respondents were asked how they were affected by client religious views and how their own religious faith and sense of spirituality affected their work with clients.

One additional hypothesis of the study was that after a number of years, response differences of both groups regarding integration of religion and spirituality would diminish because practitioners would be shaped by the concerns of their clients. This paper will focus on influence of client religious perspectives on the professional, how these perspectives affect work with clients, and ways personal religious/spiritual views may affect social work practice.

METHOD

Design

The current research used a correlational design implemented with a qualitative and quantitative survey questionnaire. The target population was graduates of a large private research university who had MSW-level preparation and a second master's degree in religion, either a MA or MDiv degree. A random sample of MSW-only graduates matched by gender and graduation year to the Dual Degree group was compiled to consider the differences in direct social work practice from those who also had university or seminary religious education.

Sample Characteristics

Respondents from the two groups did not differ significantly on most demographic data. Forty-six females and 35 males completed surveys, with nearly equal numbers of females and males among Dual Degree recipients. Respondents were primarily European American, with three African Americans, one First Nations, and one Swedish individual in the Dual Degree group. The MSW-only group contributed one Asian and two African Americans among the European Americans, so the overall sample was not very ethnically diverse. Median age across the sample was 39 years with a somewhat higher median age in the Dual Degree group (42 versus 35 years). Age range was 23 to 89 years. Median income across groups was in the $30,000 to $35,000 category (1997 figures). Nearly half (49%) of those with Dual Degrees was clergy. A religious affiliation was listed by 70% of the entire sample representing 15 denominations.

Years in social work ranged from one to 41 years with median number of years in practice at seven. MSW degrees were awarded between 1936 and 1996; religion degrees were obtained between 1951 and 1997 from eight different seminaries or universities. Of the 42 Dual Degree recipients, 17 earned the MSW and religion degree in the same year, 14 earned the religion degree first, and seven earned the MSW degree first. (Data were missing for seven.) Whether one degree was obtained first was considered a potentially significant variable for determining whether Dual Degree respondents privileged the ministerial or social work role.

Survey

The 85-item survey was designed to look at dimensions of both religion and spirituality. To provide a point of reference and commonality for random MSW-only respondents, definitions of each concept were provided. Demographic questions included both standard questions and variables unique to this population such as whether the respondent was a member of the clergy, whether the employer was a religious institution or not, and to what extent the respondent felt supported or constrained in discussing religion or spirituality with clients. Closed and open-ended questions explicitly examined respondent standpoints regarding religion and spirituality.

Procedures

This study was conducted May through July 1997 by surveying both groups of graduates described above. The Dual Degree group was located through alumni records and deans in the university divinity school and six affiliated seminaries. A record of Dual Degree students had not been widely maintained either in the social work school or by the seminaries beyond the previous four years, though university records did list some alumni who had also taken coursework at the religion school over the previous fifty years. Some alumni were listed by titles such as Rabbi, Chaplain, or Reverend that provided indications that these individuals might meet sample inclusion criteria.

All these individuals were contacted by phone to determine whether they had completed a religion or divinity degree before they were included in the sample. Recorded Dual Degree graduates were contacted and asked to provide names of other Dual Degree graduates through a snowball sampling method that also served to validate the list. The second group in the sample consisted of random graduates matched by year of graduation with a social work degree and by gender to the first group. The sample thus was skewed more heavily toward recent years when a more complete record could be constructed, though it also may be a product of a recent trend to link religion and social work study.

The survey was mailed out to 124 MSW graduates, 62 Dual Degree recipients and 62 MSW-only graduates. An introductory letter of invitation was included that contained information about the study. A second mailing was sent to nonrespondents one month later and a phone call was made in the third month. A total of 81 surveys were returned for a response rate of 65%. Two individuals in the random group were found to have seminary degrees and these cases were transferred to the Dual Degree group for data analysis. These two respondents were not replaced, so the final responses were 45 from the Dual Degree graduates and 36 MSW-only graduates. Sixty-seven respondents met the criteria of having direct practice experience, the focus of the study, though demographic data was collected on the entire sample. Complete responses were provided by 36 in the Dual Degree group and 31 in the random group, so this sample of 67 formed the basis for data analysis for the questions reported in this paper. Direct practice was self-defined.

Quantitative data was analyzed with SPSS using frequencies, chi-square, and t-tests for comparison of mean differences. Qualitative data was analyzed through the constant comparative method detailed by Strauss and Corbin (1990) where text is coded for similar categories.

RESULTS/DISCUSSION

Influence of Client Religious Views

Value in Assessment. Most survey respondents (56 out of the N of 67 fully completed surveys) discussed how they were affected by client religious views. See Table 1. A percentage of both groups (13% MSW only, 25% Dual Degree) found the religious views of clients to provide valuable information in the assessment process. "The client's religious views always let me know how I can better establish a working relationship" (MSW only, #114). "It provides information about the client's valuation of self, others, and world view. It can help define and shape areas for explora-

TABLE 1. Influence of Client Religious Views on Practitioner (N = 67)

Item	MSW only		Dual Degree		Total
	#	%	#	%	%
Views are useful in assessment: growth or defense.	4	13%	9	25%	19%
Clients are teachers, help us connect.	5	16%	3	8%	12%
I work with client beliefs.	2	6%	5	14%	10%
Fundamental views make me cautious or annoyed.	1	3%	4	11%	10%
Client religious views affect me little.	7	23%	0		10%
It piques curiosity for my own development.	0		4	11%	6%
I need to be aware of my own responses.	1	3%	2	6%	4%
I see deep spiritual hunger, religion less important.	0		2	6%	3%
I locate strengths in client religious views.	0		2	6%	3%
Other: barrier in public agency, provide religious referral.	4	13%	0		6%
Decline response.	7	23%	5	14%	18%

tion, intervention, external and internal strengths, and struggles" (MSW only, #106).

Responses by Dual Degree graduates offered a broader and contextualized description of the varied interpretative value of religion. One Dual Degree graduate (# 6) writes,

> They provide me with insight into their source of values or lack of them as well as socio-cultural understanding since religious values are intimately connected to family and family dynamics. I work in an ecumenical and multi-cultural setting, but also notice differences in generational cohorts. This present X generation has had little or no exposure to formal religious values compared to previous cohorts I deal with.

A second Dual Degree graduate relates changes in his perception,

> I used to have a good deal of discomfort with them, but now find them tremendously useful in assessing and treating clients. While I am not religious myself, I have a much greater appreciation than previously with the potentials of religion for harm and support/strength. (#14)

Personal Reactions. Other comments by Dual Degree respondents describe the personal feelings that religious discussions evoke.

- Sometimes a client's particularly bad religious experiences make me feel more cynical and skeptical. Of course I am using "good" and "bad" very subjectively as they seem to relate to the person's overall adjustment and mental health (#38).
- I often need to translate what they are saying so it has meaning for me–so I can respond appropriately. Have to slow down and stay at the level of the client. I find my own spirituality and beliefs don't match those of the general population on the surface (#54).
- We are all on the journey together. There is no one with regard to religion or spirituality who has all the answers or authority. The gifts received by me, in spiritual terms, from my clients are tremendous. My hope is that I have been at least as helpful.

A large percentage of MSW-only graduates indicated that client religious views had little effect on them (23%) or declined to respond (23%) compared with 14% of Dual Degree graduates who did not respond to this question. A few MSW-only respondents who did respond provided specific examples, such as frustration with Hispanic women who passively believe God will work things out (#62). "It gives us a point of common understanding that I have used to introduce issues that are relevant to the client's problem. It has also challenged me to appreciate the variety of religious beliefs and has expanded and deepened my own personal faith" (#70).

Though some individuals saw religious views as useful in building a therapeutic relationship, others kept it at a distance. "I respect their points of view," stated one MSW-only graduate simply (#105). Perhaps because of greater education or interest, Dual Degree graduates are more likely to notice, ask about, or be affected by client religious views.

Influence of Practitioner Religious Faith on Practice

The client/social worker relationship will optimally function reciprocally during the course of treatment. In addition to considering how client religious views affect the social worker, it is also helpful to think about the complementary pattern: how social worker religious views affect the professional relationship. See Table 2. Similar to the previous question, comparable percentages of both groups (16% MSW only; 22% Dual Degree) found their own religious background beneficial in

TABLE 2. Influence of Practitioner Religious Faith on Practice

Item	MSW only #	MSW only %	Dual Degree #	Dual Degree %	Total %
It alerts me to role of religion for clients.	5	16%	8	22%	19%
It provides guiding principles (especially service).	5	16%	6	17%	16%
I have compassion, empathy, see other as child of God.	2	6%	5	14%	10%
I have no religious faith.	5	16%	2	6%	10%
Faith centers me, gives me clarity.	1	3%	7	19%	12%
It has little influence or I keep them separate.	5	16%	1	3%	9%
I am able to be hopeful with clients.	2	6%	4	11%	9%
Spirituality is primary, more important than religion.	2	6%	3	8%	7%
I assume the role (minister or social worker) that applies.	0		5	14%	7%
I use metaphors to communicate truth.	1	3%	2	6%	4%
Declined to respond.[a]	6	20%	3	8%	13%

[a]Percents are greater than 100 as some respondents had more than one answer.

assessing the role of religion for the client. The value base of religious philosophy was also cited by both sets of respondents (16% MSW, 17% Dual Degree) for providing guidance in the treatment process. Differences begin to emerge for Dual Degree graduates in considering the personal practice of religion in social work and maintaining role distinction. The latter respondents viewed their religious grounding in an integrative manner with practice.

Faith Centers Me. The following comments were formulated by Dual Degree graduates.

- Religious faith helps me to de-center myself and listen to people within their frame (#24).
- It deepens my sense of purpose and care for my patients (#32).
- My faith fuels a sense of hope, purpose, and fulfillment (#33).
- I see my work as a ministry that helps me to treat difficult clients better (#34).
- It causes me to stay open, looking and listening with them. I am not the oracle (#51).
- It keeps me interested in the work and nurtures me in times of trial (#52).

- It grounds my talk about spiritual things in a comfortable understandable place. It encourages me to serve clients, not as objects for financial or behavioral manipulation. It provides metaphors to communicate truthfulness (#18).

Errors in Assumptions About the Meaning of Faith. Difficulty in balancing the role of clergy and social worker was addressed by several Dual Degree graduates. "I think it is constraining when the clients have an awareness of my religious practices or clergy status and bring a whole bag of role expectations for me to the client practitioner relationship" (#38). Another Dual Degree graduate demurs,

> I do not have a religious faith. Obviously, the better developed a practitioner's spirituality is, the more he/she can work imaginatively and in depth with clients in this realm. However, I think many good therapists can do "spiritual work" without calling it by that name. The shadow side can also be enacted, e.g., practitioners concerned with spirituality can err by foisting their own brands on their clients. (#14)

Concern with Focus on Religion. There was a tendency for MSW-only graduates to view religion in a constricted or concrete manner, "I can only speak intelligently with other Catholics about religion–I am not well versed in other religions" (#123). Other MSW-only respondents felt it was important to keep separate. "When working with my clients, religion is not usually the issue. I do not feel my religious faith in any way affects my work" (#88). Yet other MSW-only respondents implicitly identify the limits they set in religious discussions with clients:

> My religious connections supply the ethical and scientific principles that guide my professional behavior. They are harmonious with the ethical underpinning of social work or I would not be in the field. I see no reason why religion should be incorporated into social work curriculum or practice except as individual professionals choose. If they so choose, I think it essential that they respect client boundaries in this domain. (#86)

More individuals in the sample were willing to share responses to this question, with 20% MSW only and 8% Dual Degree graduates failing to address this.

Influence of Practitioner Spirituality on Practice

A significant percentage of respondents (16% of MSW only, 22% of Dual Degree) replied that their answer would be the same as for the previous question, indicating they do not make a clear distinction between religion and spirituality (see Table 3). Some MSW-only graduates reported helping clients let go of what they can't control using a 12-step approach. Another described spirituality as providing meaning. "My personal sense of a connection to the universe gives me a sense of confidence and satisfaction that my decision to do social work in an inner city is important" (#61). A third MSW-only respondent expresses spirituality as a process.

> My own explorations and understanding of the struggle to find spiritual guidance and grounding helps me maintain humility and compassion in my work. I try to view each encounter I have with clients as imbued with unique meaning in both my life and theirs and as an opportunity for creativity and healing. My spirituality guides my actions for healing and justice. (#92).

Dual Degree responses depicted a spectrum of ideas:

- My spirituality is the basis of my beliefs about the value and potential richness of human life. It directs the respect I feel for my clients and the humility I have in the work I do which is so painful at times (#15).
- It sensitizes me to the fact that my clients may have a very serious interest in spiritual issues, may be more serious than my own, and that I should "hear" when my clients want to talk about these matters (#38).
- My sense of spirituality adds greater depth to the practice of social work (#33).
- I make a distinction between religion (people fight wars over religion and it can be toxic) and spirituality which that part of personality that gives meaning, purpose, and goals to our life–using the more inclusive model of bio-psycho-social-spiritual concept of self. One's spirituality can be expressed in a formal and positive way through religions, but does not have to be (#6).
- I believe that life is truly difficult. I search for and cherish moments of peacefulness, a simple connectedness, a tender compassionate listening (#55).

TABLE 3. Influence of Practitioner Spirituality on Practice

Item	MSW only #	MSW only %	Dual Degree #	Dual Degree %	Total %
Spirituality provides a healing connection.	4	13%	4	11%	12%
It gives meaning to religion, adds depth.	3	10%	4	11%	10%
I use it to help others find life purpose.	3	10%	4	11%	10%
I seek to pass on my spiritual hope.	3	10%	1	3%	6%
It helps me maintain compassion.	1	3%	4	11%	7%
It sensitizes me to listen to clients.	0		5	14%	7%
I am not spiritual.	4	13%	0		6%
Spirituality forms basis of my belief, hope others find it.	0		3	8%	4%
My own spiritual growth affects my work with clients.	3	10%	0		4%
It motivates my work with poor; it is ministry.	0		2	6%	3%
I pray for clients.	0		1	3%	1%
It is the same for me as religion.	5	16%	8	22%	19%
Decline to respond.[a]	6	20%	5	14%	16%

[a]Percents are greater than 100 as some respondents had more than one answer.

Several MSW-only individuals in the sample indicated that they felt more strongly about the value of spirituality than religion. A few discussed the value of spirituality though others did not try to articulate its merit. Dual Degree respondents were more likely to address spirituality as the profound core of their religious faith and identify its capacity for personal renewal.

CONCLUSION

As in Canda and Furman's (1999) survey of NASW practitioners, both groups generally make a distinction in the terms religion and spirituality. However, clinical practice is delineated somewhat differently by individuals who possess an additional degree in religion/divinity beyond social work. These individuals tend to be more attuned to the various roles religion and spirituality may play for clients, both in their capacity to heal and also to harm. They listen to spiritual and religious stories clients relate and look for metaphorical meaning that may touch important client themes. As a group their conceptions about religion and spirituality are more complex and considered. Equally complex are the ways they choose to integrate these themes in their work with clients, both to benefit clients directly and as a source of personal renewal.

Limits of this study included too few older Dual Degree social workers to determine whether differences between the two groups narrow over time. Some clergy did not consider their work "direct practice" and opted out of the study, losing potentially important information.

Educational experience does not explain all of the difference between these two groups; there may be something unique about individuals who choose to obtain a second degree in social work or religion. Also, future research should look separately at the MSW with combinations of a MA in religion or a divinity degree which is often preparation for ordination. This study does suggest that Dual Degree graduates make an important contribution in building a holistic approach to professional social work practice. A Dual Degree does make a difference in social work.

REFERENCES

Bergin, A. E., & Jensen, J. P. (1990). Religiosity of psychotherapists: A national survey. *Psychotherapy*, *27*(1), 3-7.

Bullis, R. K. (1996). Spirituality in social work practice. Washington, DC: Taylor & Francis.

Canda, E. R. (1988). Spirituality, religious diversity, and social work practice. *Social Casework*, *69*(4), 238-247

Canda, E.R. (1997). Spirituality. In Richard L. Edwards (Ed.), *Encyclopedia of social work 19th Edition supplement* (pp. 299-309). Washington, DC: National Association of Social Workers.

Canda, E. R., & Furman, L. D. (1999*). Spiritual diversity in social work practice: The heart of helping*. New York: The Free Press.

Carroll, M. M. (2001). Conceptual Models of Spirituality. In E.R. Canda, & E. D. Smith (Eds.), *Transpersonal Perspectives on Spirituality in Social Work. Social Thought 20*(1/2) (pp. 5-23). New York: The Haworth Press, Inc.

Derezotes, D. S. (1995). Spirituality and religiosity: Neglected factors in social work practice. *Arete*, *20*(1), 1-15.

Derezotes, D. S., & Evans, K. E. (1995). Spirituality and religiosity in practice: In-depth interviews of social work practitioners. *Social Thought*, *18*(1), 39-56.

Furman, L. E. (1994). Religion and spirituality in social work education: Preparing the culturally sensitive practitioner for the future. *Social Work and Christianity: An International Journal, 21*, 103-115.

Goldberg, C. (1996). The privileged position of religion in the clinical dialogue. *Clinical Social Work Journal, 24*(2).125-136.

Herzog, S., & Russel, R. (1995). Spirituality courses in M.S.W. programs. *Society for Spirituality and Social Work Newsletter, 3*(20), 4-5.

Joseph, M. V. (1987). The religious and spiritual aspects of social work practice: A neglected dimension of social work. *Social Thought, 13*(1), 12-23.

Joseph, M. V. (1988). Religion and social work practice. *Social Casework, 60*(7), 443-452.

Marty, M. E. (1980). Social Service: Godly and godless. *Social Service Review, 54(*4), 4463-4481.

Rizer, J. M., & McColley, K. J. (1996*). Social Work and Christianity, 23*(1), 53-65.

Shafranske, E. P., & Malony, H. N. (1990). Clinical psychologists' religious and spiritual orientations and their practice of psychotherapy. *Psychotherapy, 27* (1), 72-78.

Sheridan, M. J., & Amato-von Hemert, K. (1999). The role of religion and spirituality in social work education and practice: A survey of student views and experiences. *Journal of Social Work Education, 35* (1), 125-143.

Sheridan, M. J., & Bullis, R. K. (1991). Practitioners' views on religion and spirituality. *Spirituality and Social Work Journal*, 2(2), 2-10.

Sheridan, M. J., Bullis, R. K., Adcock, C. R., Berlin, S. D., & Miller, P. C. (1992). Practitioner's personal and professional attitudes toward religion and spirituality: Issues for education and practice. *Journal of Social Work Education, 28*(2), 190-203.

Strauss, A., & Corbin, J. (1990). *Basics of qualitative research: Grounded theory procedures and techniques.* Newbury Park, CA: Sage.

Clinical Pastoral Education (CPE) and the Professional Identity of the Dual Degrees Student

Robert T. O'Gorman

SUMMARY. Students in dual degree programs have an additional task of negotiating dual professional identities. While students do this somewhat successfully, it seems they do it without any deliberate or systematic help from either their divinity or social work curricula. This article suggests that the divinity requirement for Clinical Pastoral Education (CPE) can serve as an integrating element of the curriculum and examines perceived identity blocks that may make this possible. *[Article copies available for a fee from The Haworth Document Delivery Service: 1-800-HAWORTH. E-mail address: <docdelivery@haworthpress.com> Website: <http://www.HaworthPress.com> © 2005 by The Haworth Press, Inc. All rights reserved.]*

KEYWORDS. Divinity, clinical pastoral education, identity, dual degrees, role, ministry, spirituality

---

Robert T. O'Gorman, PhD, is Professor of Pastoral Studies, and Director of Field Education, Institute of Pastoral Studies, Loyola University, Chicago, 12th Floor Lewis Towers, 820 North Michigan Avenue, Chicago, IL 60611 (E-mail: rogorma@luc.edu).

[Haworth co-indexing entry note]: "Clinical Pastoral Education (CPE) and the Professional Identity of the Dual Degrees Student." O'Gorman, Robert T. Co-published simultaneously in *Journal of Religion & Spirituality in Social Work: Social Thought* (The Haworth Social Work Practice Press, an imprint of The Haworth Press, Inc.) Vol. 24, No. 1/2, 2005, pp. 125-135; and: *Social Work and Divinity* (ed: Daniel Lee, and Robert O'Gorman) The Haworth Social Work Practice Press, an imprint of The Haworth Press, Inc., 2005, pp. 125-135. Single or multiple copies of this article are available for a fee from The Haworth Document Delivery Service [1-800-HAWORTH, 9:00 a.m. - 5:00 p.m. (EST). E-mail address: docdelivery@haworthpress.com].

http://www.haworthpress.com/web/JRSSW

Digital Object Identifier: 10.1300/J377v24n01_11

"I'll never forget it. It was my first day of CPE." The event that Doug, a first year dual degrees student, shared with his peer-learning group involved a baby who had been stillborn. The parents wanted to have a memorial service in the hospital chapel. Doug tried in vain to get an ordained minister because he felt he did not know what to do. When he found that he would need to do the service himself, he quickly prepared some things to say. However, when the nurse brought the stillborn baby into the chapel where he and the parents were, Doug found that he could not say what he had planned.

"All I could do was stand there and cry," wrote Doug. Not knowing what to expect, Doug was surprised when the nurse handed him the baby to hold. "I want you to baptize my baby. Her name is Nicole." The mother said.

Doug nodded, but he saw no water with which to baptize the baby. Almost without thinking he took a tissue, wiped the tears from the eyes of the parents and his own eyes, and touched it to the baby's head and whispered, "Nicole, I baptize you in the name of the Father, Son, and Holy Ghost. Amen" (Patton, 1990, p. 11 *adapted*).

This description comes from a dual degrees student engaging an event in a hospital where he was participating in Clinical Pastoral Education or CPE. Clinical Pastoral Education is interfaith professional education for ministry designed to provide a context to deal with the raw elements of life; to be a laboratory for the human condition. It brings theological students and ministers of all faiths (pastors, priests, rabbis, imams and others) into supervised encounters with persons in crisis. Out of an intense involvement with persons in need, and the feedback from peers and teachers, students develop new awareness of themselves as persons in terms of the needs of those to whom they minister. From theological reflection on specific human situations, they gain a new understanding of ministry and their ministerial identity. Within the interdisciplinary team process of other helping persons in the hospital, they develop skills in interpersonal and interprofessional relationships.

CPE is a required part of the curriculum of most Master of Divinity degree (MDiv) programs. This aspect of the curriculum in the dual degrees program has been a problematic requirement in terms of curricular integration. While this clinical experience parallels some first year field experiences in the Master of Social Work (MSW) curriculum, there seem to be major problems of curricular integration. Due to this failure, the student has to add another half semester of time, tuition, and effort to the dual degrees program. However, beyond this curricular burden on students, this integration failure points to a crucial issue, the dual professional identities students must negotiate as they engage the dual degrees program. This paper will examine efforts in shaping this identity.

A ministerial student who also completes a degree in social work is able to bring a greater social justice capacity to her or his parish ministry and the MSW student enrolled in the divinity degree is able to bring a worldview informed by traditions that have unambiguous values on the nature of an ultimate purpose of creation and life to his or her clinical practice. However, each of these degrees prepare persons as "social characters," Alasdair MacIntyre's term to describe persons representative of key roles in life whose work shapes our culture (MacIntyre, 1981). He argues that our identity is largely shaped by unchosen social relationships, which in turn incur unchosen obligations. Identity is a social construct, a perspective shared by a community. We are always operating, speaking, practicing within a context–community, tradition. MacIntyre points out that "when an institution–a university, say, or a farm, or a hospital–is the bearer of a tradition of practice or practices, its common life will be partly, but in a centrally important way, constituted by a continuous argument as to what a university is and ought to be or what good farming is or what good medicine is. Traditions, when vital, embody continuities of conflict" (MacIntyre, 1981, p. 206). Divinity and Social Work are traditions that are in a "continuity of conflict" as to what a dual degrees program's identity ought to be.

Do clients/parishioners encounter one or two "social characters" when they relate to a dual degrees graduate? What identity did Nicole's mother or the nurse in the hospital ascribe to Doug? Does Doug struggle with his own professional identity? Diana Garland ends her chapter, "Church Social Work: an Introduction" with an assessment of the literature, stating: "With the two degrees from different schools come two professional identities which the social worker/church leader is left to integrate and/or hold in tension with one another" (1992, p. 10). Garland suggest we have either a *dialectic* or a *duality*, oil and water or possessing the quality of being twofold. 'To integrate or hold in tension' is the fork in the road to face in the dual degrees program. Is this burden carried by the student or shared by the schools? Experiences so far suggest the former.

The first case is that of a dual degrees student working with a CPE supervisor and hospital social worker who at first jointly agreed to supervise the student. In this case the student was to participate in the group sessions with the other CPE students but visit the patients as social worker. The CPE supervisor and the Social Work supervisor planned a creative process of joint supervisory sessions with the student. However, just as the placement was ready to begin, the social worker "got cold feet" and pulled out fearing that the student would fail to keep boundaries clear between her advocacy for the needs of the patient and concern for the patient's soul. The placement fell thru and the student worked that summer in the hospital strictly as a CPE student. This necessitated an additional clinical experience as social worker and extra semester of schooling.

In the second case the student was to be under supervision of a social worker at a hospital who was willing to commit to a full joint relationship with the chaplain CPE supervisor. But this time, it was the CPE supervisor who would not entertain the idea of a cooperative placement. The chaplain claimed that to mix patient social advocacy and prayer would lessen the student's ability to be perceived by the patient as a ministerial character. He believed the student would not have the experience of being accorded clear ministerial recognition by a patient and thus not have the opportunity to experience an ascribed ministerial identity. Again, the student was required to spend an extra semester in the program.

In both these cases attempting to combine CPE and first level Social Work Field Instruction, despite the full backing and much effort on the part of both of the faculty in Divinity and Social Work, there was failure to bring about curricular integration. This impasse characterizes where we are in the dual degrees program, as Garland says "the social worker/church leader is left hold their professional identity in tension." The degrees program fails to provide a deliberate and systematic curriculum path for integration.

Do the two professions, in MacIntyre's words, have such different traditions that they demand separate and thus identities in tension? An examination of CPE may offer an integrative curricular path in face of this 'fork in the road.'

CPE History

It was at the turn of the last century that Anton Boisen (1876-1965), a congregational minister who had experienced–or better, not experienced–pastoral care during a psychiatric hospitalization became concerned that the "human factor" was ignored in the education of ministers. And so he influenced ministerial education to take into account the study of the "living human document," along with other sources of divine revelation such as scripture and tradition.

There is actually a common history that social work and ministry share regarding their movement into the hospital. A physician, Richard Cabot (1886-1939), had great concern about the specialization that emerged as hospitals became a central place health care at the beginning of the 20th century. Under these "new" circumstances patients were disrupted from their communities and the continuity of life there and isolated in a medical/scientific environment. Here they were cut off from regular attention to their social and religious needs. Dr. Cabot, who had made major contributions to medical education with case-based teaching, introduced both social work to the hospital and clinical training to seminary education. He did this in the face of and as a response to science that saw religion as antithetical to its work. His goals in clinical training of the clergy were to counteract the evils of specialization, to cultivate a devotion to the sick and to care for the growth of souls, which an encounter with life threatening circumstances provides. Cabot held that, "Religion has always been an antispecialistic force . . . (and) Priest, doctor and nurse were all one person until comparatively recent times, and the priest was that person" (Gregory, 2003, p. 15). It was only in modern times, he claimed, that there has been an unnatural separation of these professions. His efforts to unite spiritual care with medical care in the hospital were the foundations for today's attention to spirituality in health care.

In 1922 Anton Boisen took courses with Richard Cabot and in 1925 Boisen, as chaplain at Worcester State Hospital, Worcester, Massachusetts accepted the first group of four seminary students for clinical training in the hospital. Today there are over 340 centers and 670 supervisors worldwide with over 2,000 CPE students at any given time of the year.

What CPE Is

CPE is an educational process that focuses on understanding oneself in terms of motivations and human relationships, understanding of one's vocation. Central questions are, "What must I do to help?" "What most I know to help?" "What can I say to help?" and the key question, "What must I *be* to help?" (Kuether, 1953, pp. 19-20). This last is the major question because, in the human encounter, it is ultimately one's self that one brings to the other. Self-understanding and self acceptance precedes understanding and accepting the patient. Thus CPE is an educational experience in relationships. The elements of CPE are 400 hours of supervised learning made up of the actual practices of patient encounter and supervised education from those practices.

The objectives of CPE are:

- To become aware of oneself as a minister and the ways one's ministry affects persons.
- To develop the skills to provide intensive and extensive pastoral care and counseling to persons in their crises and situations.
- To understand and utilize the clinical method of learning.
- To utilize the support, confrontation and clarification of the peer group for the integration of personal attributes and pastoral functioning.
- To utilize individual and group supervision for personal and professional growth and for developing the capacity to evaluate one's ministry.
- To develop the ability to make effective use of one's religious/spiritual heritage, theological understanding, and knowledge of the behavioral sciences in pastoral ministry to persons and groups.
- To become aware of how one's attitudes, values, and assumptions, strengths and weaknesses affect one's pastoral care ministry.
- To become aware of the pastoral role in interdisciplinary relationships and work effectively as a pastoral member of an interdisciplinary team.
- To become aware of how social conditions and structures affect the lives of self and others and to effectively address these issues in ministry.
- To develop the capacity to utilize one's pastoral and prophetic perspectives in a variety of functions such as: preaching, teaching, leadership, management, pastoral care, and, as appropriate, pastoral counseling (ACPE, 2001, pp. 7-8).

Methodology

It was, in fact social work's use of case studies that became the model for CPE. The essential elements of CPE include: the actual practice of ministry to persons, detailed reporting and evaluation of that practice, pastoral supervision of that practice, a process orientation to learning, a common learning experience in a small group of peers, and an individual contract for learning consistent with the objectives of CPE. The CPE program is conducted under the auspices of an Association of Clinical Pastoral Education (ACPE)[1] certified supervisor attached to an ACPE accredited CPE center.

What happens in CPE then is an awareness of feelings, attention to the personhood of the caregiver, and a way of reflecting theologically/theoretically on experience. The emphasis is not on so much skill practice as it is on personhood and professional identity; to achieve the examination and awareness of key personhood themes (such as authority, motivation for ministry, experience of crisis, and engagement in conflict) before the student enters into ministry at the professional level. The student's theological faculty and denomination use the evaluation of the student's CPE experience to help develop and determine if the student has the personal qualities (character) and psychological readiness needed to exercise these particular dimensions of ministerial leadership.

How essentially different or unique are the aims of CPE from the aims of field instruction in social work? Is ministerial identity essentially different from social work identity, so much so that they cannot become one identity both in the student's self as well as in the eyes of the clients/parishioners, and in the view of the CPE and Social Work Field Supervisors?

Examining the dual sets of capacities needed for general work as a minister and a social worker can help determine whether there is a dualism or dichotomy between the two. One school lists their capacities for it MDiv graduate:

- *Pastoral Care*: the capacity to provide ministerial presence in daily events as well as significant moments, capability to relate to a wide spectrum of persons and needs; ability to minister effectively/initially to persons in crisis; personal wisdom along with a knowledge of community resources to assess and refer persons to appropriate additional resources.
- *Community Building*: Facility in welcoming all new and inquiring members of the faith community; assessing their need for community connection; assisting in integrating such members into various aspects of the community (social life, formation, leadership, etc.) Competency in Christian hospitality evidenced in relationship building across social status within the faith community, facilitating the relationship of the faith community with other community organizations and outreach to those in need in the local community.
- *Pastoral Administration*: capacity to lead the activities of individuals, families, groups, organizations and systems towards ownership of a common vision, facilitating overall relationships in a structure that

empowers participation in community. Fiscal capacity, organizational and managerial development.

- *Faith Formation/Education*: capacity to encourage and nurture the spiritual growth of individuals and families through the variety resources available; from large group through small group to individual processes. To encourage a deepening of one's faith, to invite a greater knowledge of one's faith tradition and other faith traditions, and to allow individuals to explore their tradition in light of current understandings and personal experience. To inform and enlighten rather than indoctrinate, to invite rather than insist, to facilitate rather than force the moving of the Spirit.
- *Ritual/Worship*: appropriation of a working knowledge of the role of ritual in socialization and social construction of meaning systems; competency in adapting existing rites to the needs of their community as well as creating rituals for the community as needs arise; ability to evaluate and critique the on-going ritual life of the community as well as to empower others for participation in this process (Master of Divinity Program, 2002, pp. 54-56).

The mission of those preparing for a divinity degree includes:

- Commitment to knowledge in the service of humanity;
- Development of the capacity for critical theological skills and ethical judgment;
- Promotion of action in the service of faith and justice;
- Integration of theological literacy, pastoral skills and personal growth;
- Response to the needs and aspirations of the world community;
- Ministry in multicultural settings. (Institute of Pastoral Studies, Loyola University Chicago, Mission Statement, 2003).

With regard to the social worker, the National Association of Social Workers (NASW) code of ethics directs that social workers promote social justice and social change with and on behalf of clients, that is, individuals, families, groups, organizations, and communities. These activities may be in the form of direct practice, community organizing, supervision, consultation, administration, advocacy, social and political action, policy development and implementation, education, and research and evaluation. Social workers seek to enhance the capacity of people to address their own needs. Social workers also seek to promote the responsiveness of organizations, communities, and other social institutions to individuals' needs and social problems. The practice of social work requires knowledge of human development and behavior; of social and economic, and cultural institutions; and of the interaction of all these factors.

Common work activities include:

- Determining people's social, emotional, and economic problems and needs;
- Providing services to address the needs of people, or referring clients for appropriate professional or community services;
- Developing resources, programs and social policies to address unmet community needs;
- Assessing, diagnosing and/or treating mental health and emotional problems (Clinical Social Work: psychotherapy and counseling);
- Working to improve social programs and health services through research and by encouraging communities and organizations to be responsive to identified needs;
- Helping people improve personal and/or social functioning by providing or referring for education, training, employment and personal growth services;
- Coordinating and working with governmental, private, civic, religious, business and/or trade organizations to combat social problems through community awareness and response programs;
- Researching, planning and developing social and health policies and programs (NASW Social Work Profession, 2003).

The mission of the social work profession is rooted in a set of core values and is the foundation of social work's unique purpose and perspective:

- Service;
- Social justice;
- Dignity and worth of the person;
- Importance of human relationships;
- Integrity;
- Competence.

This constellation of core values reflects what is unique to the social work profession. Core values, and the principles that flow from them, must be balanced within the context and complexity of the human experience:

- Social workers' primary goal is to help people in need and to address social problems;
- Social workers challenge social injustice;
- Social workers respect the inherent dignity and worth of the person;
- Social workers recognize the central importance of human relationships;
- Social workers behave in a trustworthy manner;
- Social workers practice within their areas of competence and develop and enhance their professional expertise. (NASW Code of Ethics, 2003.)

CONCLUSION

Examining the competencies and values to which both degrees aspire demonstrates duality more then dualism. Care giving and concern for the other are the hallmarks of these degrees. Their integration would seem to fit "hand and a glove." Let's go back to Doug. Is ritual baptism not a symbolic gesture of assurance to the loss of a child, which assurance the social worker conveys everyday? Can the roles of social worker and minister be seen as one role, that of a caregiver, by the parents to help them transcend what would keep them from moving on in their lives? Is hesitancy to step up to the role of caregiver shared by student as social worker and as minister?

This integration at its base takes place in the student. When a student is professionally developed in these dual capacities she or he is able to dually use them in one context or another. Experience of the identity of graduates from the dual degrees program can be described as an interplay between "noun" and "adjective." The context determines which role the noun is. Initially, one student began her work in a social service agency. There, as she worked with clients, she identified herself through her actions as a "pastoral" *social worker*. After a few years, she went to the parish and helped set up a food pantry. There she pastored parishioners with a special sensitivity to how to access social services and she identified as a social work *pastor*.

However, ought not this task of professional identity formation and integration can be deliberately and systematically part of the curriculum of the joint degrees program? The examination of CPE in light of the underlying personal care giving qualities suggests that its process can be one of the joint courses to programmatically address the integration task.

NOTE

Information on the Association of Clinical Pastoral Education can be found at the web site: *http://www.acpe.edu/*

REFERENCES

ACPE. The standards of the association for clinical pastoral education. (2001) Available: *http://www.acpe.edu/objectiv.htm* (Accessed 7/24/2003).

Garland, D. S. R. (1992). Church social work: an introduction, in Garland, D. S. R. (Ed.), *Church social work: Helping the whole person in the context of the Church.* St. Davids, PA: North American Association of Christians in Social Work.

Gregory, S. R., (2003). Growth at the edges of medical education: spirituality in American medical education. *The Pharos* (spring), 14-19.

Institute of Pastoral Studies, Loyola University Chicago, Mission statement (2003). Available: http://www.luc.edu/depts/ips/ (Accessed 7/24/2003).

Kuether, F. C., (1953) Pastoral Psychology. 4 (37) 19-20, quoted in Thomas, J. R. (2000). *A "snap hot" history (1975-2000) of the association for clinical pastoral education, inc: A celebration of the 75th anniversary of CPE: one supervisor's view.* Madison, WI: Tony's Printing.

MacIntyre, A. (1981). *After virtue*, Notre Dame, IN: University of Notre Dame Press.

Master of Divinity Program. (2002). *Field education manual*, Chicago, IL: The Institute of Pastoral Studies Loyola University.

NASW Code of Ethics. (2003) Available: http://www.socialworkers.org/pubs/code/code.asp (Accessed 7/24/2003).

NASW Social work profession (2003) Available: http://www.socialworkers.org/profession/overview.asp (Accessed 7/24/2003).

Patton, J. (1990). *From ministry to theology: pastoral action and reflection*, Nashville: Abingdon Press.

Conclusion: Current State of Social Work and Divinity Dual Degree Programs

Daniel B. Lee

SUMMARY. The first national symposium on Social Work and Divinity Dual Degree Programs was designed to examine the current state of these interdisciplinary joint degree programs from both pedagogical and practical perspectives. The underlying assumption was that a more holistic approach is needed to advance our understanding of human nature, including the dimension of spirituality and the complexity of social issues. The rationale, issues, and promise for a strong commitment on the part of participating institutions toward educating the dual degree students are reflected in the context of the symposium's theme: Building Compassionate Communities: An Integration of Theology and Social Work in Professional Education and Practice. By examining the current state of social work and divinity dual degree program at Loyola University as a case example, this paper highlights the salient ideas and reflective discussions that were emerged from the symposium. *[Article copies available for a fee from The Haworth Document Delivery Service: 1-800-HAWORTH. E-mail address: <docdelivery@haworthpress.com> Website: <http://www.HaworthPress.com> © 2005 by The Haworth Press, Inc. All rights reserved.]*

Daniel B. Lee, DSW, is affiliated with Loyola University, School of Social Work.

[Haworth co-indexing entry note]: "Conclusion: Current State of Social Work and Divinity Dual Degree Programs." Lee, Daniel B. Co-published simultaneously in *Journal of Religion & Spirituality in Social Work: Social Thought* (The Haworth Social Work Practice Press, an imprint of The Haworth Press, Inc.) Vol. 24, No. 1/2, 2005, pp. 137-155; and: *Social Work and Divinity* (ed: Daniel Lee, and Robert O'Gorman) The Haworth Social Work Practice Press, an imprint of The Haworth Press, Inc., 2005, pp. 137-155. Single or multiple copies of this article are available for a fee from The Haworth Document Delivery Service [1-800-HAWORTH, 9:00 a.m. - 5:00 p.m. (EST). E-mail address: docdelivery@haworthpress.com].

http://www.haworthpress.com/web/JRSSW

Digital Object Identifier: 10.1300/J377v24n01_12

KEYWORDS. Dual degree programs, first national symposium on social work and Divinity, curricular integration, spirituality, religion, joint program

The Council on Social Work Education listed Loyola University, Chicago as one of 14 schools that offer Divinity and Social Work dual master degrees (CSWE, 1997). Although Loyola began its dual degree program with McCormick Theological Seminary in Chicago more than three decades ago, it was in the mid 1990s when a push to widen the scope of dual degree programs came by a wave of students who were interested in combining social work practice skills and credentials with theological calling and spiritual discipline, thus increasing a holistic orientation for career and personal advancements. Recently, Loyola University School of Social Work has added three other theological schools including the Garrett-Evangelical Theological Seminary, Catholic Theological School, and Loyola University's own Institute of Pastoral Studies. In addition, students from three other denominational seminaries have pursued the dual degree program opportunities. If this trend continues, the area consortium of ten divinity schools may become the partner institutions where their students can opt to choose social work and divinity dual degree program at a graduate level. This phenomenon goes beyond the Chicago area as our nation and global society search for answers to the complexity of our societal problems (Cnaan, Boddie & Wineburg, 1999).

Currently, President Bush's plan for 'Faith-Based Initiative' has sparked interest in widening the opportunities for dual degree programs between the schools of social work and divinity while other developments are cautiously taking place from both social services sectors and religious institutions (Sherman, 2000; Sherwood, 2001; Sherwood, 2000; Sider, 2000; www.au.org/faithbased.htm; www.ngltf.org/federal/wfaith.htm; Wubenhorst & Voll, 2003). The debate on the separation of state and church is historical; nonetheless, the contemporary contexts of this old issue challenges both government and church organizations to rethink earlier basis, thus opening up other possibilities for attending to the needs of today's complex social problems. In this vein, Sider (2000) proposed five action strategies to maximize the contributions of faith-based organizations to solve today's most urgent social problems, including poverty. These are: (1) capacity building of the faith-based organizations; (2) educating the leaders of the church, government, business, media, and academia on holistic ministry; (3) analyzing and evaluating the works of faith-based organizations and academia; (4) expanding sources funding holistic ministry; and (5) re-conceptualization of public policy to support the expanded role of faith-based organizations. Others (Harper, 1999; Thornburg & Wolf, 2000) have examined the role of urban and mega churches in charitable ministries. Thornburg and Wolf (2000) found in their studies of three mega churches with regular attendance exceeding 2,000 in South Carolina that the aspect of community outreach as a part of church mission was not only preached regularly, but also structurally implemented both concrete and relational services to the un-churched in addition to benefiting their members' spiritual growth. The authors suggested that in order to increase constructive, sustainable collaboration between social workers and mega churches, it would require respectful consideration for the congregation's organizational missions and that this goes to even smaller churches (p. 147). Harper (1999) observes that successful urban churches are not only very influential in their communities for their charitable services, they are actively involved in challenging institutional inequities and in bringing about changes in public policies that keep the poor on the margin. In this light, social work education can play a vital role in preparing practitioners to incorporate field-tested models of congregational outreach ministries of care, compassion, comfort, and advocacy, while engaged collaboratively in expanding the capacities of faith-based organizations and public social service sectors toward building a more compassionate community.

The roots of social services for the care of the poor, the sick, the dispossessed, the mentally ill, and many other types of vulnerable people, of course, stemmed from the outwardly charged missions of the early church (*diakonia*). Even in the case of Japan, during the era of the post WWII reconstruction, the Yokohama Christian Community Center, built and initially supported by the North American churches, but later the local city government, began its financial aid in partnership with voluntary charity organizations in caring for the neglected people (Abe, 1976). A leading Japanese Christian social work scholar, notes:

> Since the New Delhi assembly of the World Council of Churches (1961), the Asian churches' understanding of the concept of service has been rapidly deepened. They have begun to assume the work of diakonia in the mission of the church. This has spread throughout the world. Japan is no exception. It is only hoped that the church will stand ready to serve community needs and pains as her own. (Abe, 2002, p. 4)

The variations of dual degree programs for social work and divinity exist in the structure of curricular arrangements, practica, advisement processes, and time requirements, but each program is evaluated against the CSWE accreditation standard when the program is reviewed for its accreditation. For the purpose of examining the scope of the existing MSW/MDiv Dual Degree Programs, the author introduces the Loyola Model which was reviewed in 1998 by the latest site visiting team from the Commission on Accreditation for Social Work Programs.

GOALS AND OBJECTIVES OF MSW-MDIV DUAL DEGREE PROGRAM

This program is designed for persons who have interests both in theological and pastoral studies represented by the Master of Divinity (MDiv) degree, and in the studies in clinical practice represented by the Master Degree in Social Work (MSW). The offerings of this dual degree program are jointly provided by the Loyola University's School of Social Work and Institute of Pastoral Studies. The dual degree students, like all other regular MSW students, must meet all of the academic requirements to complete their respective degrees. Each dual degree program requires that applicants apply and receive admission separately. Students must meet all admission criteria for each program and enter a prescribed structure and sequencing of courses from both programs which allows for the completion of the dual degrees one year less than it would take to complete both programs separately. For the MSW-MDiv full time students this then involves four years instead of five. The curriculum retains the core courses of both the MSW and MDiv, while electives and field work are consolidated.

The Program Goals

In addition to the general objectives of each program, the MSW-MDiv dual degree program aims at broadening the scope of interdisciplinary collaborations and the level of integration in delivery of theological/pastoral care and social work services. Students are guided by core principles to formulate their own educational experiences under the structure of faculty advisement and joint degree coordinators. The program directs students toward maximizing their learning opportunities by linking to career advancement and networking with other dual degree professionals in the fields.

The Program Objectives

The dual degree program prepares students:

- To study in an urban setting with a strong commitment to social justice and ministries of pastoral care and prophetic preaching;
- To experience diverse learning/teaching communities beyond any one discipline;
- To exposure a wide range of social and moral problems impacting individuals, families, communities, and social institutions;
- To draw upon the resources of social service agencies and church related organizations to serve the needy and the impoverished;
- To integrate social work practice values, knowledge and skills with the spiritual domains of theological education and practice;
- To gain credentials to practice clinical social work in a variety of settings where such a combined education is in demands;
- To advance interdisciplinary approaches to social policy formulation and implementations;
- To expand knowledge and skills needed to promote socioeconomic justice, professional accountability, and leadership in advocacy and services to others;
- To develop effective service delivery systems of social institutions in meeting the changing demands of diverse populations and social environments; and
- To undertake a leadership role in faith communities by guiding both professions to work collaboratively toward a more just and caring society than it is perceived to be.

The Program Evaluation

Based on the above educational objectives, the author designed an evaluative instrument to assess some empirical data from those graduates of the dual degree programs in the following four areas including: (1) curricular relevance (items 1-10); (2) graduates' satisfaction (items 11-15); (3) utilities of the dual degree program (items 16-20); and (4) graduates' narrative feedback (items 21-25). The instrument has a total of 25 items of which the first 20 items are on a five-point Likert scale, and the last five items are open-end questions. Since the initial respondents to this survey were only limited to several recent graduates (N = 4) from the Loyola's MSW/MDiv dual degree program, the detailed findings are not presented here. The overall impressions, however, made clear both positive and negative aspects of the program and the experiences graduates had. On the curricular relevance, the respondents agreed that they would recommend this same dual degree program to others who wish to pursue the similar path they have taken (item 10), and that the clinical concentration of the MSW program was congruent with the other discipline they have chosen (item 9). However, they disagreed that the integration of two disciplines was optimally achieved through the field practice (item 3), and that the academic advising was instrumental in guiding their dual degree educational planning and career development (item 8). On the graduates' satisfaction, there were mixed responses. While the majority believed that the decision they made to combine the two degree program was definitely worthwhile (item 15) and that they thought their competency in helping people has been enhanced as the results of obtaining the dual degree program (item 14), others disagreed that the dual degree credentials provided them with more choices in the job market (item 12), and that the satisfaction with what they have obtained from the dual degree program at Loyola did not change (item 11).

THE CURRICULUM DESIGN FOR THE DUAL DEGREE PROGRAM (DDP)

It is important that students understand the curriculum structure of MSW Program at Loyola when they apply for DDP. The core social work curriculum is structured into five sequences including human behavior in the social environment, practice methods, social welfare policy, social work research, and field practicum. There are two levels of instruction: foundation and advanced. In addition, students need to construct their own specialization within clinical social work at the advanced level of instruction. In order to strengthen the integration of students' dual program experiences, it is highly recommended that a seminar course on the integration of faith and social work be developed jointly by the participating schools. Two sample curriculum designs (Plan A: Block Module, and Plan B: Concurrency Module) for the DDP students are illustrated here to aid in planning of the DDP students at Loyola and the participating divinity schools.

Modules of the Alternating and Concurrent Models

The alternating module is designed for students who desire to begin their professional study of either Social Work or Divinity from the beginning. Students choose each program alternatively on an annual basis like a ping-pong match from social work to divinity and vice versa. The concurrency module, on the other hand, allows students to take their carefully planned courses from both programs simultaneously within the same academic year. Here, students take greater responsibility for integrating both classroom instruction and field practicum from the onset of their DDP. The curricular examples of these two modules that are currently used at Loyola University Chicago are introduced in the appendix.

Integration of DDP in the Practice Settings

The integration of joint disciplinary education demands more critical examinations for both pedagogical and interdisciplinary scrutiny than where we currently are. It calls for an ongoing dialogue among and between the students, field instructors, and coordinators of the Dual Degree Programs from the participating schools concerning that the major issues of theoretical and practical integration, dual identity formation, site development, supervisory qualification, spiritual formation, and evaluative criteria.

The social work internship (15 credit hours) provides the students in the dual degree program excellent opportunities for integrating theological and social work values, theories and skill development, and maximizing the resources from both disciplines and their practice settings. While they must receive social work clinical instruction from a variety of fieldwork settings under the supervision of qualified social workers, they are also expected to have a certain period of spiritual formation and pastoral field experiences under a different set of guidelines. Until such time that there are sufficient numbers of qualified dual degree field instructors who can supervise DDP students in the context of interdisciplinary practice, divinity schools need to supplement their side of field education if such is deemed necessary. There are a number of social service agencies that are faith-based and staffed by social work practitioners with divinity degrees. As time goes, the graduates from DDP become professionally matured, and ideally, they can serve as DDP field instructors. At the present time, however, students encounter a number of challenges in finding a setting that provides both spiritual and social work supervision in the context of integrating both curricula and practical dimensions of the dual degree program. To make DDP a viable option for interdisciplinary collaboration, this is one of the most urgent issues for the schools of DDP to resolve by training and recruiting DDP clinical field instructors who are equipped with integrated knowledge, skills, value orientations and commitment toward holistic care and services.

Academic Planning and Advisement

Each School appoints its DDP coordinator who oversees the integrity of the program. The appointed coordinator provides the DDP students and applicants with necessary guidance and academic planning for meaningful and effective completion of their respective degrees. Students must take responsibility in periodically scheduling with the office of DDP coordinator to design, review, and evaluate the courses of academic planning, field internship, and integration of interdisciplinary education. It is important to facilitate DDP students to develop networking and linkage with DDP alumni by cultivating such a holding environment and strengthening the integration of their new dual identity. For the continuity of coordinative services and familiarity with the progresses the DDP students are making, it is highly advisable that centralizing and monitoring the academic advisement function be maintained in the office of the DDP coordinator, thus giving the participating institutions a certain level of assurance for the integrity of the dual degree education. Periodic consultation conferences or contacts between the DDP coordinators of participating schools will enhance the spirit of collaboration and accountability to enhance the benefits of interdisciplinary education.

WHAT HAVE WE LEARNED FROM THIS SYMPOSIUM?

Issues and Challenges Being Addressed in the DDP

A number of issues that are challenging the dual degree programs in social work and divinity were highlighted at this national symposium. What we have learned the most from a close examination of the current state of DDP critically reflects the lack of integration across the fundamental theoretical bases for building an ideological synthesis. This foundational need underlies the call for curriculum integration in joint degree programs, administrative commitment, identity formation, internship development, supportive networking, and linkages to faith-based community development, and program evaluation. Some of these issues are addressed from various points of view and perspectives to strengthen academic efforts in educating dually disciplined professionals, and to respond more effectively to the demands of our time.

Challenges are still ahead of us as Canda pointed out the differences that exist between religion and social work with regards to their perspectives and theoretical bases in understanding human nature, commitment to diversity, sources of healing, sanctions for services, and role distinctions. Each discipline challenges the other in constructive ways in dual programs. Religion or religious teachings can remind social work to keep their sense of calling. It helps social workers to keep personal balance and centering on a heart of compassion and love that are necessary for transformative service. As we seek a holistic understanding of personal and social systems, religion can remind social work to recognize the divine within everyone and to regard human relationship as a reflection of the unconditional love of God for humanity. Divinity also brings an array of helping and healing strategies, techniques and supportive systems such as meditation, prayer, ritual, symbolism, and mutual supports in religious communities. Likewise, social work challenges religion to accept, help and respect all people where they are without strings attached, nor with expectation of conformity, and regardless of their diversity in all forms. Social work is often practiced in public and non-religious settings where it is not appropriate to discuss religion overtly or display one's own religious commitment. Social work blends artistry and values with scientific evidence and technical skills, thus it reminds religion to reflect critically on traditional ideas and practices about causes and solutions for human problems such as mental illness, substance abuse, and poverty. The real challenge for students in dual degree programs is how they create synergy out of connecting both social work and religion, how to balance their dual perspectives for integration, and how these connections give them profound meaning for their lives. It is an invaluable challenge to draw upon our inner and outer spiritual strength and resilience for personal growth and social justice and to increase our competence in particular skills through inspiration. Concern with differences in the religious intolerance toward liberal tradition of social work is still a challenge in the secular world of social realities and the identity-shaping reality of religion. Dual degree program students may need to go beyond their superficial level of understanding religion and psychological issues in human experience. Incompatibility issues exist between religion and social work in the areas of practice principles (client's right to self-determination, a therapeutic setting free of coercive measures, etc.) and lack of comprehensive integration of religion and social work.

Building Ideological Synthesis

Several authors addressed the ideological issues relevant to DDP. Holland hopes for both disciplines of theology and social work to engage together in dialogues, pioneering the regeneration of "an ecologically grounded spirituality of creative communion" on both local and planetary levels. He envisions the need for creating an infrastructure of professionals devoted to create "the new institutional paths of all professions" and "the new networks of electronic communications." Tyson proposes the power of care giving relationship towards developing compassionate communities in the light of Holland's hope for the postmodern transformation. She posits that "to be able to nurture compassionate communities, humans need to have a sufficient capacity for competent self-regulation–self regulation of self-worth, stable competence in choosing and pursuing one's goals and caring treatment of others." Introducing "intrapsychic humanism" which offers a therapeutic regiment to a variety of developmental and mental problems across cultures and ages, Tyson believes in the healing power of care giving relationships to which both social work and divinity are deeply committed.

Bishop Conway articulates the benefits of dually trained clinicians for their gifts in realizing both mystical dimension of spirituality and reality dimension of human nature and in responding to the wholeness of the client. In the context of his own personal faith life, Bishop Conway asserts that "the discipline of social work has been a great asset in the development of a prayer life, which is spiritually formational." While the integration of social work and faith is already taking place in the life of the Church and faith-based social services, the Catholic social teachings clearly underline the institutional commitment toward the common good globally. In the light of contemporary challenges of urbanization, globalization, corruption, drug trade and use, and ecological malaise, Bishop Conway advocates the importance of ethical education and strong relationship between social work and faith communities in overcoming the limitation of each field. We still need research to find the effect of one on the other. Harmony of social work and faith breaks down. Several critical questions were raised to move the current complexities of the dual degree programs that are caught by the schism that exists between social work and theology.

Curricula Integration

On a theoretical synthesis, Ashby identifies three common elements divinity and social work brings to the DDP: first, the common commitment to the health and well-being of individuals and communities; second, the knowledge, skills and values that bear on the human condition so as to change or transform persons and systems to better conform to the profession's vision of health and wholeness; and third, the need to be informed by other disciplines so as to effect change, transformation, health and wholeness in the most effective and comprehensive manner. He foresees the potential that dual degree programs can produce when they work more jointly to enhance the quality of educational experience and to increase their contributions toward the health and wholeness of persons and the well-being of society.

On the differing perspectives in these two professions, Ashby offers his insightful observations as follow:

> When it comes to the life of faith social work tends to be more descriptive and ministry tends to be more prescriptive. Social Work tends to recognize the presence of a transcendent other, while ministry tends to push for a kind of relationship with the transcendent other. In social work spirituality tends more to be a practice or discipline, whereas in ministry spirituality is more a way of life. Finally, in social work the life of faith is viewed as resource while in ministry the life of faith is an affirmation of faith that one lives into.

Ashby also notes the different roles social workers and ministers are taking toward the end of life:

> Social workers recognize and acknowledge the possible inclusion of spirituality as a resource for those who grieve. Making meaning at the end of life may benefit from a relationship. For ministers spirituality is a necessary part of end of life process. In ministry the pastors seeks to help the dying person and their loved ones make faith affirmations about life and death and live into those affirmation.

From the perspective of securing clients' health and wholeness, Ashby asserts that both pastoral care and psychosocial care, when they are appropriately integrated, can make much greater contributions than separately applied.

Ashby suggests four possible models of dual degrees to stimulate us to re-think their relevance. They include:

1. a ministry with social work knowledge and skills;
2. a ministry of social work;
3. social work with a religious or spiritual component; and
4. social work as ministry.

Ashby argues that these models result from a lack of clarification about the nature and intent of the dual degree program than carefully designed products of curricular integration between two disciplines. In order to advance the theoretical and practical bases for curricular integration of divinity and social work, we need more critical examinations of current curricular structure and credit arrangements of transferring courses. He, then, proposes a *joint* degree program where the joining schools hammer out the basic assumptions, values, course requirements and curricular implications of training persons in divinity and social work. This will help students to find in a mutually adopted and integrated model that reflects their joint thinking, planning, and curriculum design on the basis of common understandings. Instead of depending on the railroad track model that separates social work and divinity, a mutually influencing model of religion and social work is advocated. One creative way to facilitate integration is to require "a credit bearing course to which each school gives credit, taught by resident faculty of the two schools, whose principal aim is to assist students in the integration of divinity and social work." Essential is to have joint thinking and planning in sequencing the curriculum and to develop a maximum formation toward a holistic model of integration. Ashby recommends that field sites live out this joint identity, to have supervisors who went through dual degree programs or who hold both degrees, and to develop an integrated seminar throughout the program led by resident faculty of both disciplines for integrity of the program.

Both Northcut and Cnaan have developed courses where social work students can integrate the spiritual and psychosocial dimensions in the clinical/pastoral practices and faith-based community social services. In her newly developed course, entitled: "The Role of Religion and Spirituality in Clinical Social Work," Northcut integrates a number of salient elements in dealing with self and other from both psychological and spiritual perspectives. While examining potentially conflicting ethical issues in clinical practices, the course offers dual degree students the opportunities to foster self-awareness and personal development with a clear understanding of his or her own motives in examining religion and spirituality in the lives of clients. Although Northcut recognizes the potential clashes that can occur between practitioner beliefs, theoretical orientations, and professional beliefs, she maintains that students need to struggle in the process of reconciling the differing roles and paradoxes in beliefs. Cnaan makes a strong argument about the inclusion of religion in social work curriculum on the basis of his review of social work's roots, value stance, the relevance of religious contributions in caring and healing of people in social contexts, and empirical evidences of people's religiosity. Cnaan proposes that all social work courses, including field practica, incorporate relevant aspects of religion and to prepare social workers in both micro and macro practice to strengthen collaborative services with faith-based communities. Cnaan and others believe that schools of social work can lead the next cadre of social service providers to work with and within faith-based social service agencies and to help people who are serious about their religion to gain strength and mutual support through their religious beliefs. For many religious beliefs and practices are a source of strength, hope and survival when they face hardships such as major illnesses, job loss, traumas, or extreme poverty. Cnaan believes that out of his course teaching about organized religion in social work, not only students, faculty and field instructors were highly satisfied, but also social service agencies benefited from the integration of faith and social work.

Reflecting her own call to a *diaconate* ministry in the United Methodist denomination, which emphasis the ministry of justice and love, Crane believes that if dual degree programs seek integration, they must be joint, between faith and action, and *being* and *doing*. Dualism that exists between the clergy class and laity, church and society also must be broken so that *the diaconate* can carry out their juxtaposed ministry of social work and spiritual transformation with all needed supports from both ends.

Administrative Commitment for Better Coordination Between Partnering Programs

A number of authors have addressed the importance of coordination between the partnering programs to redress the confusion the students in the dual degree programs are currently experiencing. Course team teaching can bring more holistic perspectives for better integration, for an example, learning from dealing with a dying patient for social work vs. chaplain learning. Knowing and being integration requires balancing of both theological and social work resources. Other examples may include: lack of skills in dealing with counter transference issues or outcome measurement of ending. It is important to maintain key and co-key advisors from both disciplines for ongoing contact. The challenge is still to articulate this very issue of practice integration, how to train social work for being in the therapeutic role without losing the existing curriculum structure. In social work, currently, there is no integrative seminar for social work. Crain raises some critical questions for DDP to iron out and articulate the area of curricular integration. How to develop helpful seminar? What is its distinction? What's the commonality? Defining directions where to go. How do students discern their calls and career goals? Is it social work client or ministry parishioner or counselee? How do we respond and what's appropriate as social worker?

Identity Formulation

"Does it make a difference which school the dual degree students begin?" "How about the different orientations to supervision that both disciplines provide the student with?" Ashby and others have raised both theoretical and practical questions that demand further examinations in clarifying many challenging realms of the dual degree curricular and practical orientations. Ashby advocates for an on-going dialogue between the resident faculty of the dual degree programs to foster the identity formation process for the students; this is certainly an important task for all dual degree programs to undertake. While each discipline expects the students grasp its unique aspects of knowledge, skills and values to master, an optimal convergence can be achieved when these aspects are brought to bear in the context of wholeness and synergy in bridging gaps each discipline has failed to narrow. Concerning the formation of identity, Ashby suggests that "a student spends a concentrated period of time at both schools, rather than go back and forth. In this way the student has a chance to more successfully be formed in both disciplines."

In a close examination of the current field educational experiences of the dual degree students at Loyola, O'Gorman raises concern about the current impasse in modeling the interdisciplinary role between the field supervisors of social work and pastoral care, and also the integrative issues of personal and professional identity for students in the eyes of clients/parishioners. He notes the role of the recipients of service play in the student's identity formation, pointing to the social positions the professions of ministry and social work have respectively established in the culture. The challenge is how to mend this fragmentation. Crane affirms joint programs as vehicle to overcome dualism as she welcomes the newly emerging order of the deacon in the United Methodist Church which embodies the interrelationship of the church and world.

Joint thinking and planning is so essential that the institutions that run dual degree programs should provide the necessary structure and resources towards achieving a higher level of synergistic integration and recognition of gifts students bring into the joint education and practice. On the other hand, Northcut believes that "the task of forming a healthy dual professional identity relies on students having the transitional space to create the complexity needed." The tension that has existed for a long time is due, in part, to the schism between theology and social work from the differences of language and philosophical bases despite key shared concepts such as human dignity and social justice.

Supportive Networking

The very question of integration raised by other authors is raised again by Crane in the context of supportive systems from the ecclesiastical bodies that supervise programs of formation and education for *the diaconate* who need money, time, and emotional supports to complete the dual degree programs. Without such supports, the students will continue to experience isolation, displacement, and split over the course of their dual degree education. Bishop Conway affirms the importance of institutional supports towards dual degree students so that they are equipped with value commitment, needed professional knowledge and skills, and a sense of mission.

Some other issues that need to be addressed in future symposia include: maintenance of professional practice boundaries, tension between secular and spiritual realms, dual degree program evaluation, development of joint field sites and supervision, linkages to faith based communities, and the like. Voices of DDP students and alumni need to be systemically incorporated as feedback for strengthening the program structure, joint advisement and guides, curricular integration, field sites development, and coordination between the partnering programs for joint course development and collaborative research. There is a delicate boundary for DDP interns in dealing with clients' confidentiality issue and religiosity. This reaffirms the position many other writers' emphasis on holistic approach to meet the needs of clients. Like the courses, developed by Northcut and Cnaan, to incorporate the role of religion and faith-based communities in expanding the repertoires of social work, writers advocate: (1) comprehensive integration of coursework and field education with development of joint courses and discussion groups; (2) continuity of student advisement being handled by the DDP coordinators of the partnering programs to handle issues of cross coordination and advising students; (3) development of joint field sites for dual degree students with clear guidelines for program requirements, mutual expectations, goals and boundaries, and goal-oriented structure of learning and evaluation; and (4) support and accountability of field sites administration and staff to uphold the philosophy, values and requirements of each dual degree programs.

CONCLUSION

In the light of the current trends that bring a new generation of social work and divinity students to dual degree programs, the opportunities to deepen their sense of calling and to broaden their integrative perspectives of practice challenge both educators and learners with many complex tasks associated with the uncharted pathways ahead of them. This first national symposium and its contributors met its first challenge to examine the current state of social work and divinity dual degree programs in the United States. The voices of concerns and promises were heard with critical ears and hopeful visions. A number of current dual degree students and recent graduates of dual degree programs who actively participated in the dialogical discourse at this symposium felt encouraged and recognized their shared role in shaping the future of dual degree programs toward a higher level of curricular integration, structural coherence, cultivation of supportive networks, and ideological synthesis.

Nelson-Becker, in her recent comparative study of those social work practitioners with and without religious education, affirms that "Dual Degree graduates make an important contribution in building a holistic approach to professional social work practice." She, then, concludes in her presentation that:

> . . . these individuals tend to be more attuned to the various roles religion and spirituality may play for clients, both in their capacity to heal and also to harm. They listen to spiritual and religious stories clients relate and look for metaphorical meaning that may touch important client themes. As a group their conceptions about religion and spirituality are more complex and considered. Equally complex are the ways they choose to integrate these themes in their work

with clients, both to benefit clients directly and as a source of personal renewal.

Where do we go from here? The next challenge is not so much with what to do but as much as how to become. Mother Theresa once made a keen observation with regards to social workers: They tend to be obsessed with doing rather than being with those who have spiritual needs for our connected presence in the midst of human suffering and alienation. As many authors reflected upon the convergent values of social work and theology with regard to human worth and dignity, growth and resourcefulness, relationship and social justice, each discipline can join the other toward maximizing the realization of those shared values, visions, skills and resources. Social contexts and faith traditions are by products of humanity's quest for meaning, thus, clients and practitioners can make an optimal choice in determining the most relevant course of meeting their existential quest whatever substantive elements therein–be it psychological, social or spiritual.

In ending this segment, let the collective prayers offered by the dual degree students who served as volunteers at the symposium site be heard and echoed locally and globally:

Morning Prayer

(April 20, 2002)

God, we praise you and give you thanks
for your continued grace and the gift of this time together.
We ask that you help us to grow in faith as one community
And make all of us instruments of your peace.
Fill us today with your divine wisdom.
Illuminate our hearts as well as our minds.
Bring us into closer fellowship with you, Lord, and with each person here today.
Help us to learn from each other–and from you.
Creator God, we humbly offer all that we are
And all that we do into your hands.
Forgive us when we fail to be signs
of your steadfast love in this broken world.
Creator of the Universe–Power and Force that bonds all that Exist.
Give us the "Way"–we so desperately seek.

May our efforts to understand each other
be successful and lasting.
O, God, we pray for unity,
Give guidance from above.
In our differences unite us
In the circle of your love.
Take our many ways of working-blend the colors of each soul
Into the beauty of a rainbow.
Give us life, Lord.
Make us whole.
We ask that you guide our feet and strengthen us
For the journey to which you have called us.
May our time together now be inspired by your presence;
That we might grow in faith and serve you better.
We pray these things trusting fully
In your perfect love and wisdom. AMEN.

REFERENCES

Abe, S. (1976). *A Christian view of and response to social need in Japan.* Address presented on the occasion of the 30th anniversary of the Yokosuka Christian Community Center, Yokosuka, Japan.

______(2002). *The changing face of Christian social work in Japan.* A paper prepared for the memorial symposium in the honor of the late Dr. Dock Joon Kim, a founding Korean Christian Social Welfare Education in Korea, Seoul, Korea.

Cnaan, R. A., Boddie, S. C., & Wineburg, R. J. (1999). *The newer deal: Social work and religion in partnership.* New York: Columbia University Press.

Council on Social Work Education (1997). *The handbook of MSW Programs.* Alexandria, VA: CSWE.

http://www.ngltf.org/federal/wwfaith.htm. George W. Bush's Faith Based Initiatives.

http://www.au.org/faithbased.htm. Americans united for separation of church and state: President Bush's faith-based initiatives: An American's united response.

Harper, N. (Ed.), (1999). *Urban churches, vital signs: Beyond charity toward justice.* Grand Rapids, MI: Eerdmans.

Sherman, A. (2000). Tracking charitable choice: A study of the collaborations between faith-based organizations and the government in providing social services in nine states. *Social Work and Christianity, 27*(2): 112-129.

Sherwood, D. (2000). *Tracking charitable choice: A study of the collaborations be tween faith-based organizations and the government in providing social services.* Botsfold: the North American Association of Christians in Social Work.

______(2001). Integrating faith and social work practice: Evangelism. *Social Work and Christianity, 29*(1):1-12.

Sider, R. (2000). Maximizing the contribution of faith-based organizations to solve today's most urgent social problems. *Social Work and Christianity, 27*(1): 71-79.
Thornburg, G.. & Wolf, T. (2000). Megachurch involvement in community ministry. *Social Work and Christianity, 27*(2): 138-149.
Wubbenhorst, W.. & Voll, M. N. (2003). Enough about leveling the playing field: What's the playing field? *Social Work and Christianity, 30*(1): 14-37.

Index

